Placenta Accreta Spectrum

Sherif A. Shazly • Ahmed A. Nassr
Editors

Placenta Accreta Spectrum

Basic Science, Diagnosis, Classification and Management

Springer

Editors
Sherif A. Shazly
Department of Obstetrics and Gynecology
Leeds Teaching Hospitals NHS Trust
Leeds, UK

Ahmed A. Nassr
Department of Obstetrics and Gynecology
Baylor College of Medicine
Houston, TX, USA

ISBN 978-3-031-10349-0 ISBN 978-3-031-10347-6 (eBook)
https://doi.org/10.1007/978-3-031-10347-6

This Springer imprint is published by the registered company Springer Nature Switzerland AG
The registered company address is: Gewerbestrasse 11, 6330 Cham, Switzerland

Contents

Contributors

Mahmoud A. Abdel-Aleem Department of Obstetrics and Gynecology, Assiut University, Assiut, Egypt

Maryam Abdelkarim Obstetrics and Gynecology Department, Faculty of Medicine, Alexandria University, Alexandria, Egypt

Mostafa H. Abouzeid Women Health Hospital, Assiut University, Assiut, Egypt

Department of Obstetrics and Gynecology, Assiut University, Assiut, Egypt

Dema Adwan Department of Obstetrics & Gynecology, Damascus University, Damascus, Syria

University Hospital of Obstetrics and Gynecology, Damascus University, Damascus, Syria

Islam A. Ahmed Faculty of Medicine, Assiut University, Assiut, Egypt

Mhd Ali Alabdulrazak Faculty of Medicine, Damascus University, Damascus, Syria

Mustafa Albokai Faculty of Medicine, Damascus University, Damascus, Syria

AlBatool M. AlMahdy Faculty of Medicine, Assiut University, Assiut, Egypt

Grace Ariani Department of Anatomical Pathology, Dr. Soetomo Academic General Hospital, Universitas Airlangga, Surabaya, Indonesia

Rozi Aditya Aryananda Dr. Soetomo Academic General Hospital, Universitas Airlangga, Surabaya, Indonesia

Mohamed I. Ateya Department of Obstetrics and Gynecology, South Valley University, Qena, Egypt

Nicolás Basanta Fernández Hospital and School of Medicine, 1° Anatomy Chair, University of Buenos Aires, Buenos Aires, Argentina

Michael A. Belfort Department of Obstetrics and Gynecology, Baylor College of Medicine and Texas Children's Hospital, Houston, TX, USA

Alekhya Chintamani Department of Obstetrics and Gynaecology, Canberra Health Services, Canberra, ACT, Australia

Ayman S. Dawood Obstetrics and Gynecology Department, Faculty of Medicine, Tanta University, Tanta, Egypt

Deniz Dirik Medical Faculty, Department of Obstetrics and Gynecology, Van Yuzuncu Yil University, Van, Turkey

Gena M. Elassall Faculty of Medicine, Assiut University, Assiut, Egypt

Nashwa Anwar Eltaweel Department of Obstetrics and Gynaecology, University Hospitals of Coventry and Warwickshire, Coventry, UK

Elif Yagmur Erdem Department of Obstetrics and Gynecology, Ege University School of Medicine, Izmir, Turkey

Ahmet Mete Ergenoglu Department of Obstetrics and Gynecology, Ege University School of Medicine, Izmir, Turkey

Karin A. Fox Department of Obstetrics and Gynecology, Baylor College of Medicine and Texas Children's Hospital, Houston, TX, USA

Ahed Hamed Department of Obstetrics & Gynecology, Damascus University, Damascus, Syria

Al Zahrawi Maternity Hospital, Damascus, Syria

Ahmed Y. Hefnawy Department of Obstetrics and Gynaecology, The Northern Care Alliance NHG group, Oldham, Manchester, UK

Ismet Hortu Department of Obstetrics and Gynecology, Ege University School of Medicine, Izmir, Turkey

Onur Karaaslan Medical Faculty, Department of Obstetrics and Gynecology, Van Yuzuncu Yil University, Van, Turkey

Erbil Karaman Medical Faculty, Department of Obstetrics and Gynecology, Division of Gynecologic Oncology, Van Yuzuncu Yil University, Van, Turkey

Boon Lim Department of Obstetrics and Gynaecology, Canberra Health Services, Canberra, ACT, Australia

Australian National University, Canberra, ACT, Australia

Ana Paula Machado Serviço de Ginecologia e Obstetrícia, Centro Hospitalar São João, Porto, Portugal

Tatiana B. Makukhina Federal State Budgetary Educational Institution of Higher Education "Kuban State Medical University" of the Ministry of Healthcare of the Russian Federation, Faculty of Postgraduate Education, Department of Obstetrics, Gynecology and Perinatology, Krasnodar, Russia

Marina Moucho Serviço de Ginecologia e Obstetrícia, Centro Hospitalar São João, Porto, Portugal

Ahmed A. Nassr Department of Obstetrics and Gynecology, Baylor College of Medicine and Texas Children's Hospital, Houston, TX, USA

Álbaro Nieto-Calvache Placenta Accreta Spectrum Clinic, Fundación Valle del Lili, Cali, Colombia

José M. Palacios-Jaraquemada CEMIC University Hospital and 1° Anatomy Chair, School of Medicine, University of Buenos Aires, Buenos Aires, Argentina

Universitas Airlangga, Surabaya, Indonesia

Grigory A. Penzhoyan Federal State Budgetary Educational Institution of Higher Education "Kuban State Medical University" of the Ministry of Healthcare of the Russian Federation, Faculty of Postgraduate Education, Department of Obstetrics, Gynecology and Perinatology, Krasnodar, Russia

Pedro Viana Pinto Serviço de Ginecologia e Obstetrícia, Centro Hospitalar São João, Porto, Portugal

Faculdade de Medicina, Universidade do Porto, Porto, Portugal

Nourah Al Qahtani Obstetrics and Gynecology Department, Imam Abdulrahman Bin Faisal University, Dammam, Kingdom of Saudi Arabia

Ahmad A. Radwan Faculty of Medicine, Assiut University, Assiut, Egypt

Bahram Salmanian Department of Obstetrics and Gynecology, Baylor College of Medicine and Texas Children's Hospital, Houston, TX, USA

Esraa G. Sayed Faculty of Medicine, Assiut University, Assiut, Egypt

Ahmed S. Sedik Faculty of Medicine, Assiut University, Assiut, Egypt

Sohum C. Shah Department of Obstetrics and Gynecology, Baylor College of Medicine and Texas Children's Hospital, Houston, TX, USA

Scott A. Shainker New England Center for Placental Disorders, Beth Israel Deaconess Medical Center, Boston, MA, USA

Department of Obstetrics, Gynecology, and Reproductive Biology, Harvard Medical School, Boston, MA, USA

Alireza A. Shamshirsaz Department of Obstetrics and Gynecology, Baylor College of Medicine and Texas Children's Hospital, Houston, TX, USA

Sherif A. Shazly Department of Obstetrics and Gynecology, Leeds Teaching Hospitals NHS Trust, Leeds, UK

Omima T. Taha Obstetrics and Gynecology Department, Faculty of Medicine, Suez Canal University, Ismailia, Egypt

Sarah Tounsi Department of Obstetrics and Gynecology, Baylor College of Medicine and Texas Children's Hospital, Houston, TX, USA

Chapter 1
History of Placenta Accreta Spectrum

Nashwa Anwar Eltaweel and Ahmed Y. Hefnawy

The placenta accreta spectrum is a broad-spectrum pathology related to the abnormally deeply invading and abnormally adherent placental tissues through the uterine wall. Many theories tried to explain the reason behind the pathology; however, the most popular theory is the destruction of the decidual lining either by the previous caesareans, curettage, infection, IVF, or myomectomy; simply any disruption of the endometrial lining can predispose to the deeper implantation of the placenta through the underlying myometrial layer. The degree of this adherence to or through the myometrium will further classify the severity of the pathology [1].

With the rising rates of caesarean section deliveries, it is believed that it was associated with the new emerging pathology "placenta accreta spectrum" despite lacking strong evidence to support this theory [2]. By searching the literature, we noted that, in 1885, the first suspected pathologically adherent placenta was described when Macdonald described a case of a suspected adherent placenta following a prolonged vaginal birth, where some cotyledons were retained intrauterine following vaginal delivery; the patient was managed conservatively by opiate for pain control and ergot as an ecbolic to enhance uterine activity. The cotyledons were retained for days and passed spontaneously as they could not be removed manually; however, the patient had postpartum sepsis [3].

In 1927, **S Foster**, from Montreal hospital in Canada, reported "a case of placenta accreta". The patient had a vaginal breech delivery for a dead fetus. After delivery, he could not deliver the placenta despite a trial of manual removal under

N. A. Eltaweel (✉)
Department of Obstetrics and Gynaecology, University Hospitals of Coventry and Warwickshire, Coventry, UK
e-mail: Nashwa.eltaweel@uhcw.nhs.net

A. Y. Hefnawy
Department of Obstetrics and Gynaecology, The Northern Care Alliance NHG group, Oldham, Manchester, UK

S. A. Shazly, A. A. Nassr (eds.), *Placenta Accreta Spectrum*,
https://doi.org/10.1007/978-3-031-10347-6_1

general anaesthesia. Due to the repeated attempts to deliver the placenta, suspected tearing of placenta tissues occurred and was followed by excessive bleeding needing an emergency hysterectomy [4]. Dr. Foster suggested the rough incidence of 1 in 8000 cases in his maternity department after performing a 6-year survey in Montreal General Hospital. Also, he mentions a similar case reported previously by **Andrews** in 1924: the patient who had a previous history of endometritis and curettage had a vaginal delivery followed by an adherent placenta, which is resistant to separation and complicated by severe postpartum haemorrhage bleeding [5]. However, Andrews could not find a cleavage plane to separate the placenta, so he delivered the placenta in pieces and packed the uterus for 36 hours. However, he mentioned that a hysterectomy would have been the safest and more logical management. In both cases, the obstetricians noted that they could not obtain a cleavage line, and on pathology assessment, the absence of decidua was noted. In Andrew's report, he mentioned a previously reported literature review of 22 cases of suspected placenta accreta by **Dietrich** in 1922 [5].

In 1937, **Irving and Hertig** reported a cohort of 18 cases of placenta accreta, where they gave the first description of what is currently known as a morbidly adherent placenta. They described it clinically as a partial or total adherence of the placenta to the uterine wall and described it histologically as a presumed partial or total absence of the decidua basalis [6]. They also included the previously called deeper placentation and probable placenta increta and percreta under the general title of placenta accreta. They presumed a prevalence of 1 in 1965 cases among the population tested in Boston Lying-in Hospital and 1 in 30,000 in the United States [7].

The placenta accreta incidence has risen dramatically over the past 50 years, from 1 in 4000 deliveries in the 1970s to around 1 in 500 recently. This alarming figure was notoriously attributed to the increasing worldwide rate of caesarean sections [8].

Various terms have been used to describe the placenta accreta spectrum: morbidly adherent placenta, placenta adhesive disorder, abnormally invasive placentation, abnormally adherent, abnormal placental adherence, and advanced invasive placentation and abnormal myometrial invasion [9]. That is why a priority came for a standard universal terminology of the placenta accreta spectrum for the overall pathology like an umbrella with definite subtypes underneath for better determination of the extent of the disease and easier description of the pathology for the communication between the physicians [10].

Lukes et al. in 1966 presented a theory that a different nomination structure should be used. They recommended using placenta accreta vera if the decidua is absent but the villi did not penetrate through the myometrium, use placenta accreta if it invades the myometrium, and use percreta if it invades the serosa. Also, they advised adding the description of partial or total to describe the extent of the pathology [11]. The normal placental tissues are invasive tissues, so adding the title abnormal to the terminology invasive placenta is advisable [12].

Recently, it has been recommended to use the universal terminology of the placenta accreta spectrum and aim for specification of the subtype (accreta, percreta, or increta) [10]. Those three subtypes came from the pathological diagnosis or assessment of the extent of the disease, so accreta means that the placental villi are adherent to the myometrium, increta if it invades the myometrial layer, and percreta when the villi invade the serosal layer as well. Following that, many publications reporting and reviewing placenta accrete spectrum became available. However, a recommendation for a final joint diagnosis of clinical, radiological, and pathological diagnosis should always be achieved [13]. The European Working Group on Abnormally Invasive Placenta (EW-AIP) strongly recommended using the general title AIP (abnormally invasive placenta) until a final diagnosis is reached following histopathological examination [14].

References

1. Eshkoli T, Weintraub AY, Sergienko R, Sheiner E. Placenta accreta: risk factors, perinatal outcomes, and consequences for subsequent births. Am J Obstet Gynecol. 2013;208(3):219. e1-.e7
2. Collins SL, Chantraine F, Morgan TK, Jauniaux E. Abnormally adherent and invasive placenta: a spectrum disorder in need of a name. Ultrasound Obstet Gynecol. 2018;51(2):165.
3. MacDonald KN. How to prevent septicaemia in cases of morbidly adherent placenta. Br Med J. 1885;1(1268):779.
4. Forster DS. A case of placenta accreta. Can Med Assoc J. 1927;17(2):204–7.
5. Andrews CJ. Report of a case of retained placenta, clinically placenta accreta. J Am Med Assoc. 1924;82(22):1780.
6. Irving F. A study of placenta accreta. Surg Gynecol Obstet. 1937;64:178–200.
7. Jauniaux E, Silver RM, Matsubara S. The new world of placenta accreta spectrum disorders. Int J Gynecol Obstet. 2018;140(3):259–60.
8. Booker W, Moroz L. Abnormal placentation. In Seminars in perinatology 2019 (43, 1, pp. 51–59). WB Saunders.
9. Jauniaux E, Collins SL, Jurkovic D, Burton GJ. Accreta placentation: a systematic review of prenatal ultrasound imaging and grading of villous invasiveness. Am J Obstet Gynecol. 2016;215(6):712–21
10. Jauniaux E, Collins S, Burton GJ. Placenta accreta spectrum: pathophysiology and evidence-based anatomy for prenatal ultrasound imaging. Am J Obstet Gynecol. 2018;218(1):75–87.
11. Luke RK, Sharpe JW, Greene R. Placenta accreta: the adherent or invasive placenta. Am J Obstet Gynecol. 1966;95(5):660–8.
12. Collins SL, Chantraine F, Morgan TK, Jauniaux E. Abnormally adherent and invasive placenta: a spectrum disorder in need of a name. Ultrasound Obstet Gynecol. 2018;51(2):165–6.
13. Fox H. Placenta accreta, 1945–1969. Obstet Gynecol Surv. 1972;27(7):475–90.
14. Collins S, Ashcroft A, Braun T, Calda P, Langhoff-Roos J, Morel O, et al. Proposal for standardized ultrasound descriptors of abnormally invasive placenta (AIP). Wiley Online Library; 2016. p. 271–5.

Chapter 2
Epidemiology of Placenta Accreta Spectrum: A Comprehensive Review of Current Evidence

Alekhya Chintamani and Boon Lim

Introduction

Once considered a rare condition, the diagnosis and management of placenta accreta spectrum (PAS) is receiving significant attention due to increased prevalence worldwide [1–3]. If not suspected at time of delivery attempts, manually extracting the placenta can lead to major obstetric haemorrhage, peripartum hysterectomy and potential complex surgery with resultant morbidity and mortality [4]. The risk is particularly high in invasive cases where chorionic villi have invaded into surrounding pelvic organs and vasculature [5, 6], frequently leading to early delivery [7–9].

Earlier theories hypothesised that the condition developed due to a primary defect in the biological function of the trophoblast leading to excessive invasion of placental tissue into the myometrium [10, 11]. Subsequently, the prevailing hypothesis is that the defect lies in the endometrium-myometrium interface, usually due to a prior hysterotomy, leading to a failure of normal decidualisation in the corresponding uterine area. This allows for the anchoring chorionic villi to morbidly adhere to the myometrium and for further trophoblastic invasion [10].

Increasing incidence of placenta accreta spectrum disorders has been largely attributed to increasing caesarean section rates observed worldwide [4]. However, other aetiologies such as advanced maternal age and fertility and gynaecological procedures have been implicated in its etiopathogenesis. Understanding its

A. Chintamani
Department of Obstetrics and Gynaecology, Canberra Health Services, Canberra, ACT, Australia

B. Lim (✉)
Department of Obstetrics and Gynaecology, Canberra Health Services, Canberra, ACT, Australia

Australian National University, Canberra, ACT, Australia
e-mail: Boon.Lim@act.gov.au

S. A. Shazly, A. A. Nassr (eds.), *Placenta Accreta Spectrum*,
https://doi.org/10.1007/978-3-031-10347-6_2

prevalence and risk factors allows for earlier diagnosis and planned multidisciplinary management which is essential in reducing unexpected complications and morbidity.

This chapter will outline the prevalence of placenta accreta spectrum worldwide and its increasing trend globally, as well as risk factors contributing to disease epidemiology.

Definition and Terminology

Though descriptions of likely placenta accreta date as far back as the sixteenth century, the condition was first formally described in a case series published by Irving and Hertig in 1937 [12, 13]. They used a clinical definition of the abnormal adherence of the placenta to the uterine wall, or histologically as the complete or partial absence of the decidua basalis. At that time, invasive forms of placenta accreta were not encountered in their cohort of patients with the majority having unscarred uteri. Luke et al. [14] subsequently redefined the condition as a group of abnormally adherent or invasive placental disorders with subdivisions representing the level of placental invasion. These now form the accepted grading of placenta accreta (anchoring villi adhering to superficial myometrium), placenta increta (villi penetrate the myometrium) and placenta percreta (anchoring villi penetrate through full-thickness myometrium and extend into surrounding organs). These conditions are now collectively known as placenta accreta spectrum.

Ideally, histopathological definitions would provide a gold standard for diagnosis of the condition; however, this is not always possible nor accurate. The degrees of invasion may coexist in the same clinical scenario as they may range from being focal in one area to extensive invasion in another part of the uterus. Myometrial fibres have been found in the basal plates of normal placenta [15], the decidua becomes thinner with age and is not uniform [10], and in some cases histopathological assessment is unable to be performed. Therefore, clinical diagnosis and description remain the most feasible global definition. This variability has sometimes contributed to inaccurate diagnoses. It is known that accurate and consistent antenatal diagnosis allows for an improved multidisciplinary approach to management with improved maternal and fetal outcomes. International consensus panels have convened to discuss terminology, diagnosis and reporting of invasive placental disorders in order to address clinical and histopathological variation in reporting [16, 17]. The respective Expert Groups devised a consensus approach to the ultrasound diagnosis as well as a new detailed grading system based on findings at both laparotomy and histopathology. Both systems aim to produce uniformity in diagnosis, reporting and reproducibility of data in future literature.

Despite these clinical definitions, there remains significant heterogeneity in interpretation and classification of abnormal placentation in literature leading to variation in reported incidence and prevalence. A number of descriptive terminologies such as abnormally invasive placenta (AIP) or morbidly adherent placenta

(MAP) have also been used to describe this group of conditions. Placenta accreta spectrum (PAS) is an umbrella term that recognises the continuum on which many adherent placental conditions lie and will be used for the remainder of this chapter.

Incidence and Increasing Trend Globally

A significant challenge in obtaining epidemiological data on placenta accreta spectrum disorders lies in the inconsistencies in terminology and diagnostic criteria used. Table 2.1 illustrates the range of reported PAS incidence and significant heterogeneity that can be observed across described studies by population studied and definitions used.

Incidence from most developed countries in the last decade range from 0.017% to 0.106% [3, 9, 18–22].

The majority of studies were performed in single tertiary teaching hospitals. Given that many of these hospitals were in major capital cities and were likely referral centres for high-risk pregnancies, their numbers may not reflect incidence in the wider population. Zeng et al. [23] found that up to two thirds of women with PAS disorders in their study came from women in rural areas. Bailit et al. [20] conducted their study over 25 hospitals across Canada, excluding Quebec, and found a statistically significant difference in prevalence of PAS amongst them ranging from 0 to 1:197 births. Furthermore, given that several studies had a large proportion of patients that did not have an antenatal diagnosis of PAS (even up to 70% of patients in the NOSS study conducted by Thurn et al. [3]), this may reflect an underestimate of PAS cases that occur in these outer metropolitan hospitals who were not referred to tertiary centres for multidisciplinary care.

A number of countries utilised their own nationwide health database collection or adopted the World Health Organization International Classification of Diseases (ICD) coding systems to circumvent these limitations. However, the ninth edition of ICD did not contain a code for placenta accreta. This was updated in ICD-10 and endorsed by the World Health Organization in 1990 and was accepted globally at differing times with the United States not implementing ICD-10 until 2015. This affected study periods covered and the ability to compare trends over time. Mehrabadi et al. [18], for example, only began collecting routine diagnostic information on their Canadian population in 2009 and therefore conducted their analysis following this time.

Studies utilised a mix of clinical, histopathological and imaging-based diagnosis of PAS in reporting the incidence of PAS. Higher incidences of PAS ranging from 0.137% to 0.636% were reported when broader case definitions were set such as the inclusion of placentas that did not separate at or immediately after delivery, as well as morbidly adherent placenta [18, 20, 24, 25].

In comparison, when stricter definitions were used, an almost fourfold lower incidence of PAS was reported. For example, Higgins et al. [26] defined PAS as an abnormally adherent placenta requiring a peripartum hysterectomy and

Table 2.1 Prevalence of placenta accreta worldwide and their corresponding study characteristics

Study name	Years studied	Study type	Patient population	Definition	Incidence n (%)
Farquhar et al [21]	2010–2012	Prospective case control	Australia/New Zealand: Bi-national data 667, 936 AMOSS study	Imaging/clinical/histological Diagnosed as placenta accreta by either antenatal imaging, at operation, or histological specimens	295 (0.044%)
Baldwin et al [33]	2003–2012	Retrospective cohort	Australia: 922, 925 births New South Wales data only	ICD-10-Australian modification code for placenta accreta, increta and percreta	2285 (0.248%)
Michikawa et al [24]	2005–2010	Retrospective cohort	Japan: 40,573 births Western districts of Japan in tertiary-level hospitals	National database codes for placenta accreta—Defined as abnormal adherence of the placenta to the uterus	258 (0.636%)
Vinograd et al [79]	1988–2010	Retrospective cohort	Israel: Single tertiary hospital unit. 239,640 births	ICD-9 code for abnormally adherent placenta found at caesarean section or needing surgical/manual removal post-vaginal delivery + histopathological diagnosed cases	551 (0.230%)
Jauniaux et al [80]	1982–2018	Systematic review and metanalysis	29 studies from global mix of nations, retrospective/prospective studies 5,719,992 births	Articles published in English only. MeSH terms: Placenta accreta/increta/percreta + abnormally invasive placenta, morbidly adherent placenta and major placenta previa	7001 (0.17%)
Higgins et al [26]	1975–2010	Retrospective cohort	Ireland: Single tertiary unit, women who had one or more previous caesarean sections, 157,162 births in multiparous women	Placenta that is abnormally adherent to the uterus sufficient to require a peripartum hysterectomy and confirmation by histology	1 (0.004%) 1975–1979 15 (0.025%) 2003–2010
El Gelany et al. [31]	2017–2018	Prospective cohort	Egypt: Single tertiary hospital, total births not stated	Women diagnosed with PAS prenatally via imaging	102 (0.91%)
Cal et al [22]	2009–2018	Retrospective cohort	Portugal: Single tertiary hospital 23,707 births	Database + ICD-9 coding with histological confirmation	15 (0.063%)
Brennan et al [27]	2000–2013	Retrospective cohort	Australia single tertiary hospital 111,056 births	Histological diagnosis of placenta accreta/increta/percreta	101 (0.091%)

Thurn et al [3]	2009–2012	Prospective	Nordic countries (Denmark, Finland, Iceland, Norway and Sweden) 605,362 births NOSS study	ICD-10 coding + International database + mailed in surveys Defined as abnormally invasive placenta found at caesarean section or vaginal delivery leading to laparotomy and blood transfusion needed secondary to AIP.	205 (0.034%)
Mehrabadi et al [18]	2009–2010	Retrospective cohort	Canada: 570,537 births	Canadian health system ICD coding Placenta accreta as a broad term including placental adhesion to the uterine wall/musculature/surrounding organs	819 (0.144%)
Bailit et al [20]	2008–2011	Prospective cohort	USA: Teaching hospitals (22/25 teaching hospitals) 115,502 births	Included morbidly adherent placenta defined as placenta not separating with ease from the uterine wall at or immediately after delivery. No histopathological confirmation. Cases diagnosed antenatally were checked for postnatal confirmation	158 (0.137%)
Upson et al [19]	2005–2010	Retrospective case control	Ireland: 403,602	ICD-10—Australian modification code for morbidly adherent placenta at discharge coding	Overall incidence 357 (0.088%) 2005–0.079% 2010–0.106%
Fitzpatrick et al [9]	2010–2011	Prospective population-based study	221 UK hospitals 798,634 births UKOSS study	Clinicians asked to mail in their cases each month. Histological diagnosis of placenta accreta/increta/percreta + abnormally adherent placenta requiring active management including conservative approaches leaving the placenta in situ (clinical and pathological)	134 (0.017%)

(continued)

Table 2.1 (continued)

Study name	Years studied	Study type	Patient population	Definition	Incidence n (%)
Guleria et al [34]	2001–2010	Retrospective	India: Single tertiary hospital 100,892 births	Ultrasound/MRI diagnosis + clinical diagnosis + histological diagnosis	Overall 56 (0.056%) 2001–2005 17 (0.031%) 2005–2010 39 (0.083%)
Esh-Broder et al [66]	2004–2009	Retrospective cohort	Israel: Single tertiary teaching hospital 25,193 births	Clinical cases that were proven on histopathology	42 (0.167%)
Wu et al [81]	1982–2002	Retrospective	USA, single teaching hospital 64,359 births	Histopathology OR clinical diagnosis	121 (0.188%)
Gielchinsky et al [2]	1990–2000	Retrospective cohort	Israel: Single hospital 34,450 births	Clinical or histological criteria	310 (0.900%)
Kayem et al. [67]	2013–2015	Prospective population-based study	France: 176 representative maternity hospitals 520,114 births PACCRETA study	Clinical or histological definition Clinical: Partial or impossible manual removal of placenta and no cleavage plane between uterus and placenta	249 (0.048%)
Zeng et al. [23]	2007–2016	Retrospective cohort	China: Single tertiary hospital 26,214 births	Clinical diagnosis at caesarean delivery and histological specimens post-hysterectomy	302 (1.152%)
Kyozuko et al. [25]	2011–2014	Prospective cohort	Japan: National data across 15 regional hospitals 90,554 births	Clinical and histological diagnosis	202 (0.223%)
Ornaghi et al. [82]	2014–2016	Prospective population-based study	Italy: 458,995 births	Used the Italian Obstetric Surveillance System (ItOSS)	384 (0.084%)

confirmation by histopathology resulting in an incidence rate of 0.004–0.025% over their study period. Thurn et al. [3] defined PAS as an abnormally invasive placenta found at caesarean section or vaginal delivery leading to laparotomy and blood transfusion, which has an incidence rate of 0.034%.

In addition to variations of clinical definitions, studies reporting histological and image-based diagnoses may have overestimated and underestimated incidence of PAS in their populations.

For example, Bailit et al. [20] showed that 30% of their PAS cases were managed conservatively without hysterectomy. This accounts for a large proportion of unaccounted PAS cases in studies that used a purely histopathological definition such as that conducted by Brennan et al. [27]

Farquhar et al. [21] conducted an Australasian-based prospective study that included cases of PAS diagnosed by antenatal imaging, clinically at time of operation, and through histopathology. Up to 36% of their case population were diagnosed by antenatal imaging, and they noted the possibility of an overestimation of cases. Inclusions of image-based diagnoses in incidence calculations may not be reproducible in low-income countries that do not have access to appropriate imaging modalities. Although magnetic resonance imaging (MRI) has been demonstrated to be an excellent imaging modality in the detection of PAS [28], two systematic reviews and meta-analyses have found that the diagnostic value of ultrasound imaging and MRI in detecting placenta accreta spectrum is similar [29, 30].

Three studies reported exceptionally high rates of PAS ranging from 0.9% to 1.152%. On further analysis, Gielchinsky et al. [2] used a broad case definition of difficult-to-remove placenta and even included cases of retained products of conception post-birth requiring curettage—both of which may have contributed to overestimation of PAS incidence in their population. El Gelany et al. [31] conducted their study in Egypt and found a PAS rate of 0.91% amongst their cohort. In their study population, 82% had greater than or equal to two previous caesarean sections, one-third had a previous history of placenta praevia, and 60% had a parity greater than or equal to 3—all known risk factors in the development of PAS. Indeed, Egypt has been listed in the top five countries worldwide for highest caesarean section rates [32]. Likewise, Zeng et al. [23] reported the highest incidence of PAS in their national study at 1.152%, though noted 93.7% of women with PAS had a previous history of caesarean section. Following the introduction of the universal two-child policy in 2015, China saw a marked increase in primary caesarean section rates and of women returning for elective repeat caesarean sections.

Though it may not be possible to estimate an accurate global incidence or rise in incidence, data from studies showing trends in fixed populations has shown a rise in incidence of PAS.

Baldwin et al. [33] found over their 10-year study period that the incidence of PAS increased significantly from 20.6 to 26.9 per 10,000 deliveries in their Australian population. Likewise, Guleria et al. [34] compared the incidence of PAS in their Indian population over two time periods between 2001 and 2010 and found a rise in incidence from 0.031% to 0.083%. Zeng et al. [23] noted an increase from 0.1% in 2007–2008 to 2.1% in 2015–2016 in their Chinese cohort. Higgins et al.

[26] also noted a significant rise in incidence from 0.004% in 1975–1979 to 0.025% in 2003–2010 in their Irish population—an almost two and a half-fold increase. This was consistent with Upson et al.'s [19] study in Ireland who noted a rise from 0.079% in 2005 to 0.106% in 2010. All five studies attributed this rise to a corresponding rise in national caesarean section rates.

Of note is data lacking from African countries. Global caesarean section rates are highest in Latin America and the Caribbean (42.8%) and lowest in sub-Saharan Africa (5.0%). A systematic review and random effect metanalysis conducted by Cresswell et al. [35] investigating prevalence of placenta praevia worldwide showed significant heterogeneity in prevalence reported with geographic region being the only statistically significant variable. The highest reported cases were amongst Asian studies and the lowest were amongst Sub-Saharan African studies. It would be interesting to investigate whether this translates to incidence of PAS globally.

Morbidity and Mortality

Though comparatively uncommon, PAS remains a major contributor of maternal morbidity in the developed world [6, 36, 37]. Maternal mortality rates in the setting of known PAS disorders have been reported as high as 7% [38] increasing up to 30% in the absence of antenatal diagnosis [39]. Despite greater than 35 years of ultrasound diagnosis of placenta accreta abnormalities, there remain no global screening protocols. The recent international consensus proforma that was developed for ultrasound reporting in suspected abnormally invasive placenta aims to standardise the diagnostic approach [17]. A study conducted in India found that the majority of PAS-related cases of maternal mortality were in patients who had not had an antenatal diagnosis of PAS. They attributed lack of access to specialist surgeons and intensive care units, as well as blood transfusion products, as contributing risk factors in mortality [34]. Further studies in high-income countries revealed that up to half of all PAS disorders remain undiagnosed prenatally [3, 20]. Antenatal detection and multidisciplinary team management allows for planned delivery and has been shown to reduce maternal peripartum haemorrhage and morbidity [40, 41].

Risk Factors

Major risk factors for placenta accreta spectrum include the following:

- Previous caesarean delivery.
- Placenta praevia, especially with a history of previous caesarean section.
- Uterine surgery, including endometrial curettage, manual removal of placenta.
- Advanced maternal age.
- Assisted reproductive techniques, particularly in vitro fertilisation.
- History of placenta accreta spectrum in a previous pregnancy.

Caesarean Section

There is strong epidemiological evidence linking the global rise in caesarean section rates and incidence of PAS [3, 26, 42–45]. Caesarean sections were introduced in modern obstetric practice at the end of the nineteenth century and were rarely performed before the 1920s [46]. The advent of antibiotics and improved anaesthetic and surgical techniques reduced the morbidity and mortality associated with caesarean sections [46]. In their 1937 study, Irving and Hertig had only 1 out of 18 cases with a history of previous caesarean section, and they estimated the incidence of placenta accreta to be 1 in 30,000 deliveries [13]. The last 25 years has seen a marked increase in the rates of caesarean section worldwide with the highest rates seen in Latin America and the Caribbean (42.8%) and eastern Asia (33.7%) [32]. This increase has been paralleled with an almost linear increase in the rates of PAS detected worldwide [3, 26, 42, 43, 45]. Table 2.2 illustrates the changes in caesarean delivery rates and placenta accreta spectrum disorders over time. The change in PAS disorders often lag behind an increase in caesarean section rates by 1 to 2 decades [47].

The proposed pathogenic process is surgical damage that leads to an interruption in the endometrium and smooth muscle layers of the myometrium. This results in local hypoxia, and unlike epithelial layers of the endometrium and uterine peritoneum that heal by regeneration, the myometrium heals through formation of collagen and other connective tissues [48]. This results in increased blastocyst attachment to the scar as well as increased trophoblastic invasion [49]. Indeed, uterine scar defects have been found to be present on ultrasound in 20–65% of women with previous caesarean sections [50].

A direct association between the increase in PAS and the increase in caesarean deliveries is reported in epidemiological studies. Silver et al. [42] demonstrated the link between the number of caesarean sections and the risk of PAS, placenta praevia and hysterectomy (Table 2.3). The Nordic Obstetric Surveillance Study found that the risk of invasive placentation increases sevenfold after one prior caesarean sect. [7] and a summary odds ratio (OR) of 1.96 (95% CI 1.41–2.74) for placenta accreta spectrum after a caesarean section in a meta-analysis of 5 cohorts and 11 case-control studies. Stratification for the number of previous caesarean sections showed the OR for placenta accreta spectrum in a subsequent pregnancy ranging between 8.6 (95% CI 3.536–21.078) [37] and 17.4 (95% CI 9.0–31.4) for two previous caesarean sections and 55.9 (95% CI 25.0–110.3) for three or more caesarean sections [51]. With this knowledge in mind, women should be counselled that a higher number of caesarean deliveries are associated with a higher chance of PAS.

Studies are now investigating modifiable risk factors with caesarean section technique. A study conducted in Japan found a higher rate of PAS when a prior hysterotomy was closed with continuous rather than interrupted sutures [52]. One study found a higher risk of placenta accreta in a subsequent pregnancy when a woman had a prior history of primary caesarean delivery without labour compared to after onset of labour [53], whilst another found an inverse relationship between

Table 2.2 Changes in cesarean delivery rate and placenta accreta spectrum (PAS) disorder prevalence over time

Author	Type of study	Country of origin	Cesarean delivery rate period A (years)	Cesarean delivery rate period B (years)	PAS disorders period A (years)	PAS disorders period B (years)
Wu et al. [15] (2005)[a]	Matched case-control study	USA	12.5% (1982)	23.5% (2002)	0.38 per 1000 births (1982)	1.88 per 1000 births (2002)
Higgins et al. [20] (2013)[b]	Cohort study	Ireland	4.1% (1975)	20.7% (2010)	1.65 per 1000 births after prior cesarean (2003)	2.37 per 1000 births after prior cesarean (2010)
Morlando et al. [18] (2013)[c]	Cohort study	Italy	17% (1970s)	64% (2000s)	1.20 per 1000 births after prior cesarean (1976–1978)	3.11 per 1000 births after prior cesarean (2000s)
Cheng and Lee [24] (2015)[d]	Cohort study	Hong Kong	19.5% (1999–2003)	27.1% (2009–2013)	0.17 per 1000 births after prior cesarean (1999–2003)	0.79 per 1000 births after prior cesarean (2009–2013)

Ref: Jauniaux E, Chantraine F, Silver RM, Langhoff-Roos J, Diagnosis FPA, Management Expert Consensus P. FIGO consensus guidelines on placenta accreta spectrum disorders: Epidemiology. Int J Gynaecol Obstet. 2018;140(3):265–73

[a]Total prevalence 0.19% (121 cases of PAS disorders out of 64,359 deliveries during the study period)

[b]Total prevalence 0.01% (36 cases of PAS disorders out of 275,121 deliveries during the study period)

[c]Total prevalence 0.16% (50 cases of PAS disorders out of 30,491 deliveries during the study period)

[d]Total prevalence 0.05% (39 cases of PAS disorders out of 81,497 deliveries during the study period)

Table 2.3 Association between number of caesarean sections and risk of placenta accreta, placenta praevia and hysterectomy

Number of previous caesarean section(s)	Number of women	Number of women with placenta accreta	Chance of placenta accreta if placenta praevia	Number of hysterectomies
0	6201	15(0.24%)	3%	40 (0.65%)
1	15,808	49 (0.31%)	11%	67 (0.42%)
2	6324	36 (0.57%)	40%	57 (0.9%)
3	1452	31 (2.13%)	61%	35 (2.4%)
4	258	6 (2.33%)	67%	9 (3.49%)
5	89	6 (6.74%)	67%	8 (8.99%)

Reference: Silver RM, Landon MB, Sorokin Y, Miodovnik M, Carpenter M, Peaceman AM, et al. Maternal morbidity associated with multiple repeat cesarean deliveries. Obstetrics and gynecology (New York 1953). 2006;107(6):1226–32 interpregnancy interval and development of PAS [54]. Though there is low level evidence to support these associations, they provide an avenue for further research into the impact surgical technique may have.

Comparatively fewer large-scale studies have focused on non-previa- and non-caesarean section-related risk factors in the incidence of PAS.

Placenta Praevia

Placenta praevia is one of the most predictive risk factors in the development of PAS and at one stage was considered necessary in its diagnosis [51, 55]. A systematic review reported an increase in the incidence of PAS of 3.3–4.0% in women with placenta praevia and no previous caesarean delivery [42]. The risk of developing placenta praevia following caesarean section has been well demonstrated, increasing up to 50% following a single caesarean section and up to two-folds higher compared with women who have had two previous vaginal deliveries [56]. The combination of placenta praevia and previous caesarean section confers the highest risk group in the development of PAS [12, 18, 42, 49]. Incidence of placenta accreta in these patients with placenta praevia have been noted as high as 1/9 [51] to 1/16 [57]. The UK case-control study using the UK Obstetric Surveillance System found that the incidence of placenta accreta spectrum increases from 1.7 per 10,000 women overall to 577 per 10,000 in women with both a previous caesarean section and placenta praevia, respectively [9]. A large multicentre cohort study conducted in the USA demonstrated an increased risk of accreta in women with placenta praevia with each subsequent caesarean section. This suggests that there may be tropism of the blastocyst for the uterine scar tissue [49]; hence, clinicians should have increased suspicion in these patients.

Advanced Maternal Age

Advanced maternal age has been linked with a higher risk of maternal morbidity and adverse perinatal outcomes as well as placenta accreta [19, 21, 23, 58, 59]. Usually defined as 35 years or older, this association is a relevant modern-day risk factor with a rise in delayed childbearing noted in developed countries [59–62]. This association may represent an altered hormonal or implantation environment leading to increased rates of PAS [49]. However, it is also important to note there may be confounding factors such as increasing parity, greater history of prior gynaecological procedures, increased rates of placenta praevia and an accumulation of environmental and behavioural risk factors that play a role in incidence of PAS in these populations [63, 64]. The role of advanced maternal age in abnormal placentation should be considered when providing reproductive counselling.

Assisted Reproductive Technologies

As women choose to delay pregnancy, utilisation of assisted reproductive technologies (ART) to assist with fertility has increased. Approximately 1.9% of all births in the USA are conceived using ART and this rate is increasing [65]. The link between ART and PAS was first discovered in 2011 [66], and since then several studies have reconfirmed this association [25, 66–68]. Within the field of IVF, cryopreserved embryo transfer during hormone replacement cycle has shown the strongest association in the development of placenta accreta when compared to fresh embryo transfer, spontaneous pregnancies and natural cycle transfers [68, 69]. Theories on its etiopathogenesis include altered endometrial receptivity, defective trophoblastic invasion, and the need for a thin endometrium prior to transfer [70]. It is important to consider the overlap between maternal factors that contribute to infertility and risk factors for PAS such as advanced maternal age and previous uterine surgery. However, even after controlling for known risk factors, IVF has been shown to be an independent risk factor [69, 71].

Previous Gynaecological History

Whilst a history of caesarean delivery is a significant risk factor, other causes of surgical trauma to the integrity of the uterine endometrium and/or superficial myometrium, such as those following uterine curettage, manual removal of the placenta, postpartum endometritis or myomectomy, have been inconsistently associated with PAS in subsequent pregnancies. The UKOSS study showed that the adjusted odds ratio for placenta accreta spectrum after previous uterine surgery is 3.40 (95% CI 1.30–8.91) [9]. The development of placenta accreta spectrum has also been reported in women with no surgical history but presenting with some form of uterine pathology, such as a bicornuate uterus, adenomyosis, submucous fibroids and myotonic dystrophy [72].

Previous Obstetric History

A history of prior placenta accreta or adherent placenta presents as an increasingly encountered modern-day risk factor. Conservative management to preserve fertility and reduce morbidity associated with peripartum hysterectomy has garnered interest in literature with studies looking into obstetric outcomes in subsequent pregnancies. Baldwin et al. [73] found a PAS recurrence rate of 38/689 (5.5%, 95% CI 3.9–7.5%) compared with their population prevalence of 25.5/10000. This was consistent with Gielchinsky et al. [2] and Sentilhes et al. [74] who both found higher risks of PAS in subsequent deliveries. The current hypothesis attributes conservative management with worsening endometrial disease through further surgical intervention or risks of infection [74]. In fact, moderate to severe quantities of synechiae have been observed in women with a history of PAS and may be the contributing factor in its subsequent development [74, 75].

Management

Management options are dependent on the availability of different diagnostic and supportive modalities. There is a significant geographic variability in the approach to the management of PAS which vary from expectant management, use of methotrexate, uterine sparing procedures, hysterectomy and interventional radiology. The Global Placenta Accreta Spectrum Survey (GPASS) study was based on responses from 136 centres around the world that manage PAS. Although geographic variations in management approaches are noted worldwide, there is an overwhelming consistency of strong adherence to many existing PAS care guidelines, with some local practices demonstrating clear deviations. There is a need for further research into diagnostic and management approaches to ensure an evidence-based approach to definitions and management strategies [76].

Conclusion

There remain remarkable variations in the definition and approaches to diagnosis and management of PAS across the world. This makes it challenging to establish the true incidence of the condition. However, what is clear is that modern obstetric practice and lifestyle changes such as delayed conception, rising maternal age, assisted reproductive techniques and rising rates of caesarean deliveries are important contributory factors. With these factors in mind, there should be heightened awareness and index of suspicion, especially when a woman presents with a past history of a caesarean section, placenta praevia or uterine surgery. Antenatal detection and timely diagnosis of abnormal placentation are vital in reducing unexpected morbidity. It allows for patient counselling, multidisciplinary approach and preoperative scheduling [64, 77, 78], factors which are vital for improved maternal and fetal outcomes.

References

1. Bowman ZS, Eller AG, Bardsley TR, Greene T, Varner MW, Silver RM. Risk factors for placenta accreta: a large prospective cohort. Am J Perinatol. 2014;31(9):799–804.
2. Gielchinsky Y, Rojansky N, Fasouliotis SJ, Ezra Y. Placenta accreta—summary of 10 years: a survey of 310 cases. Placenta. 2002;23(2–3):210–4.
3. Thurn L, Lindqvist PG, Jakobsson M, Colmorn LB, Klungsoyr K, Bjarnadóttir RI, et al. Abnormally invasive placenta—prevalence, risk factors and antenatal suspicion:

results from a large population-based pregnancy cohort study in the Nordic countries. BJOG. 2016;123(8):1348–55.
4. Silver RM, Branch DW. Placenta Accreta Spectrum. N Engl J Med. 2018;378(16):1529–36.
5. Hubinont C, Mhallem M, Baldin P, Debieve F, Bernard P, Jauniaux E. A clinico-pathologic study of placenta percreta. Int J Gynaecol Obstet. 2018;140(3):365–9.
6. Marcellin L, Delorme P, Bonnet MP, Grange G, Kayem G, Tsatsaris V, et al. Placenta percreta is associated with more frequent severe maternal morbidity than placenta accreta. Am J Obstet Gynecol. 2018;219(2):193. e1-e9
7. Chantraine F, Nisolle M, Petit P, Schaaps JP, Foidart JM. Individual decisions in placenta increta and percreta: a case series. J Perinat Med. 2012;40(3):265–70.
8. Seet EL, Kay HH, Wu S, Terplan M. Placenta accreta: depth of invasion and neonatal outcomes. J Matern Fetal Neonatal Med. 2012;25(10):2042–5.
9. Fitzpatrick KE, Sellers S, Spark P, Kurinczuk JJ, Brocklehurst P, Knight M. The management and outcomes of placenta accreta, increta, and percreta in the UK: a population-based descriptive study. BJOG. 2014;121(1):62–70. discussion -1
10. Jauniaux E, Collins S, Burton GJ. Placenta accreta spectrum: pathophysiology and evidence-based anatomy for prenatal ultrasound imaging. Am J Obstet Gynecol. 2018;218(1):75–87.
11. Jauniaux E, Jurkovic D. Placenta accreta: pathogenesis of a 20th century iatrogenic uterine disease. Placenta. 2012;33(4):244–51.
12. Carusi DA. The placenta accreta spectrum: epidemiology and risk factors. Clin Obstet Gynecol. 2018;61(4):733–42.
13. Irving C, Hertig AT. A study of placenta accreta. Surg Gynecol Obstet. 1937;64:178–200.
14. Luke RK, Sharpe JW, Greene RR. Placenta accreta: the adherent or invasive placenta. Am J Obstet Gynecol. 1966;95(5):660–8.
15. Jauniaux E, Bhide A, Burton GJ. Pathophysiology of Accreta. 1st ed. CRC Press; 2017. p. 13–28.
16. Hecht JL, Baergen R, Ernst LM, Katzman PJ, Jacques SM, Jauniaux E, et al. Classification and reporting guidelines for the pathology diagnosis of placenta accreta spectrum (PAS) disorders: recommendations from an expert panel. Mod Pathol. 2020;33(12):2382–96.
17. Alfirevic Z, Tang AW, Collins SL, Robson SC, Palacios-Jaraquemada J. Ad-hoc international AIPEG. Pro forma for ultrasound reporting in suspected abnormally invasive placenta (AIP): an international consensus. Ultrasound Obstet Gynecol. 2016;47(3):276–8.
18. Mehrabadi A, Hutcheon JA, Liu S, Bartholomew S, Kramer MS, Liston RM, et al. Contribution of placenta accreta to the incidence of postpartum hemorrhage and severe postpartum hemorrhage. Obstet Gynecol. 2015;125(4):814–21.
19. Upson K, Silver RM, Greene R, Lutomski J, Holt VL. Placenta accreta and maternal morbidity in the Republic of Ireland, 2005-2010. J Matern Fetal Neonatal Med. 2014;27(1):24–9.
20. Bailit JL, Grobman WA, Rice MM, Reddy UM, Wapner RJ, Varner MW, et al. Morbidly adherent placenta treatments and outcomes. Obstet Gynecol. 2015;125(3):683–9.
21. Farquhar CM, Li Z, Lensen S, McLintock C, Pollock W, Peek MJ, et al. Incidence, risk factors and perinatal outcomes for placenta accreta in Australia and New Zealand: a case-control study. BMJ Open. 2017;7(10):e017713.
22. Cal M, Nunes C, Clode N, Ayres-de-Campos D. Placenta accreta overlying a caesarean section scar: a 10-year experience in a Tertiary-Care Centre in Portugal. Acta Medica Port. 2021;34(4):266–71.
23. Zeng C, Yang M, Ding Y, Duan S, Zhou Y. Placenta accreta spectrum disorder trends in the context of the universal two-child policy in China and the risk of hysterectomy. Int J Gynaecol Obstet. 2018;140(3):312–8.
24. Michikawa T, Morokuma S, Yamazaki S, Fukushima K, Kato K, Nitta H. Exposure to air pollutants during the early weeks of pregnancy, and placenta praevia and placenta accreta in the western part of Japan. Environ Int. 2016;92-93:464–70.

25. Kyozuka H, Yamaguchi A, Suzuki D, Fujimori K, Hosoya M, Yasumura S, et al. Risk factors for placenta accreta spectrum: findings from the Japan environment and Children's study. BMC Pregnancy Childbirth. 2019;19(1):447.
26. Higgins MF, Monteith C, Foley M, O'Herlihy C. Real increasing incidence of hysterectomy for placenta accreta following previous caesarean section. Eur J Obstet Gynecol Reprod Biol. 2013;171(1):54–6.
27. Brennan DJ, Schulze B, Chetty N, Crandon A, Petersen SG, Gardener G, et al. Surgical management of abnormally invasive placenta: a retrospective cohort study demonstrating the benefits of a standardized operative approach. Acta Obstet Gynecol Scand. 2015;94(12):1380–6.
28. Tinari S, Buca D, Cali G, Timor-Tritsch I, Palacios-Jaraquemada J, Rizzo G, et al. Risk factors, histopathology and diagnostic accuracy in posterior placenta accreta spectrum disorders: systematic review and meta-analysis. Ultrasound Obstet Gynecol. 2021;57(6):903–9.
29. D'Antonio F, Iacovella C, Palacios-Jaraquemada J, Bruno CH, Manzoli L, Bhide A. Prenatal identification of invasive placentation using magnetic resonance imaging: systematic review and meta-analysis. Ultrasound Obstet Gynecol. 2014;44(1):8–16.
30. Meng X, Xie L, Song W. Comparing the diagnostic value of ultrasound and magnetic resonance imaging for placenta accreta: a systematic review and meta-analysis. Ultrasound Med Biol. 2013;39(11):1958–65.
31. El Gelany S, Mosbeh MH, Ibrahim EM, Mohammed M, Khalifa EM, Abdelhakium AK, et al. Placenta Accreta Spectrum (PAS) disorders: incidence, risk factors and outcomes of different management strategies in a tertiary referral hospital in Minia, Egypt: a prospective study. BMC Pregnancy Childbirth. 2019;19(1):313.
32. Betran AP, Ye J, Moller AB, Souza JP, Zhang J. Trends and projections of caesarean section rates: global and regional estimates. BMJ Glob Health. 2021;6:6.
33. Baldwin HJ, Patterson JA, Nippita TA, Torvaldsen S, Ibiebele I, Simpson JM, et al. Maternal and neonatal outcomes following abnormally invasive placenta: a population-based record linkage study. Acta Obstet Gynecol Scand. 2017;96(11):1373–81.
34. Guleria K, Gupta B, Agarwal S, Suneja A, Vaid N, Jain S. Abnormally invasive placenta: changing trends in diagnosis and management. Acta Obstet Gynecol Scand. 2013;92(4):461–4.
35. Cresswell JA, Ronsmans C, Calvert C, Filippi V. Prevalence of placenta praevia by world region: a systematic review and meta-analysis. Tropical Med Int Health. 2013;18(6):712–24.
36. Grobman WA, Bailit JL, Rice MM, Wapner RJ, Reddy UM, Varner MW, et al. Frequency of and factors associated with severe maternal morbidity. Obstet Gynecol. 2014;123(4):804–10.
37. Fonseca A, Ayres de Campos D. Maternal morbidity and mortality due to placenta accreta spectrum disorders. Best Pract Res Clin Obstet Gynaecol. 2021;72:84–91.
38. O'Brien JM, Barton JR, Donaldson ES. The management of placenta percreta: conservative and operative strategies. Am J Obstet Gynecol. 1996;175(6):1632–8.
39. Aggarwal R, Suneja A, Vaid NB, Yadav P, Sharma A, Mishra K. Morbidly adherent placenta: a critical review. J Obstet Gynaecol India. 2012;62(1):57–61.
40. Tikkanen M, Paavonen J, Loukovaara M, Stefanovic V. Antenatal diagnosis of placenta accreta leads to reduced blood loss. Acta Obstet Gynecol Scand. 2011;90(10):1140–6.
41. Chantraine F, Braun T, Gonser M, Henrich W, Tutschek B. Prenatal diagnosis of abnormally invasive placenta reduces maternal peripartum hemorrhage and morbidity. Acta Obstet Gynecol Scand. 2013;92(4):439–44.
42. Silver RM, Landon MB, Sorokin Y, Miodovnik M, Carpenter M, Peaceman AM, et al. Maternal morbidity associated with multiple repeat cesarean deliveries. Obstet Gynecol (New York 1953). 2006;107(6):1226–32.
43. Morlando M, Sarno L, Napolitano R, Capone A, Tessitore G, Maruotti GM, et al. Placenta accreta: incidence and risk factors in an area with a particularly high rate of cesarean section. Acta Obstet Gynecol Scand. 2013;92(4):457–60.
44. Cook JR, Jarvis S, Knight M, Dhanjal MK. Multiple repeat caesarean section in the UK: incidence and consequences to mother and child. A national, prospective, cohort study. BJOG. 2013;120(1):85–91.

45. Creanga AA, Bateman BT, Butwick AJ, Raleigh L, Maeda A, Kuklina E, et al. Morbidity associated with cesarean delivery in the United States: is placenta accreta an increasingly important contributor? Am J Obstet Gynecol. 2015;213(3):384. e1-11
46. Jauniaux E, Grobman W. Textbook of caesarean section. Oxford: Oxford University Press; 2016.
47. Jauniaux E, Chantraine F, Silver RM, Langhoff-Roos J, Diagnosis FPA, Management Expert Consensus P. FIGO consensus guidelines on placenta accreta spectrum disorders: Epidemiology. Int J Gynaecol Obstet. 2018;140(3):265–73.
48. Jauniaux E, Burton GJ. Pathophysiology of placenta accreta spectrum disorders: a review of current findings. Clin Obstet Gynecol. 2018;61(4):743–54.
49. Ali H, Chandraharan E. Etiopathogenesis and risk factors for placental accreta spectrum disorders. Best Pract Res Clin Obstet Gynaecol. 2021;72:4–12.
50. van der Voet LF, Bij de Vaate AM, Veersema S, Brolmann HA, Huirne JA. Long-term complications of caesarean section. The niche in the scar: a prospective cohort study on niche prevalence and its relation to abnormal uterine bleeding. BJOG. 2014;121(2):236–44.
51. Zaki ZM, Bahar AM, Ali ME, Albar HA, Gerais MA. Risk factors and morbidity in patients with placenta previa accreta compared to placenta previa non-accreta. Acta Obstet Gynecol Scand. 1998;77(4):391–4.
52. Sumigama S, Sugiyama C, Kotani T, Hayakawa H, Inoue A, Mano Y, et al. Uterine sutures at prior caesarean section and placenta accreta in subsequent pregnancy: a case-control study. BJOG. 2014;121(7):866–74. discussion 75
53. Kamara M, Henderson JJ, Doherty DA, Dickinson JE, Pennell CE. The risk of placenta accreta following primary elective caesarean delivery: a case-control study. BJOG. 2013; 120(7):879–86.
54. Wax JR, Seiler A, Horowitz S, Ingardia CJ. Interpregnancy interval as a risk factor for placenta accreta. Conn Med. 2000;64(11):659–61.
55. Clark SL, Koonings PP, Phelan JP. Placenta previa/accreta and prior cesarean section. Obstet Gynecol. 1985;66(1):89–92.
56. Getahun D, Oyelese Y, Salihu HM, Ananth CV. Previous cesarean delivery and risks of placenta previa and placental abruption. Obstet Gynecol. 2006;107(4):771–8.
57. Usta IM, Hobeika EM, Musa AA, Gabriel GE, Nassar AH. Placenta previa-accreta: risk factors and complications. Am J Obstet Gynecol. 2005;193(3 Pt 2):1045–9.
58. Pinheiro RL, Areia AL, Mota Pinto A, Donato H. Advanced maternal age: adverse outcomes of pregnancy, a meta-analysis. Acta médica portuguesa. 2019;32(3):219–26.
59. Laopaiboon M, Lumbiganon P, Intarut N, Mori R, Ganchimeg T, Vogel JP, et al. Advanced maternal age and pregnancy outcomes: a multicountry assessment. BJOG. 2014;121(Suppl 1):49–56.
60. Hamilton BEPD, Martin JA, Osterman MMHS, Curtain SMA. Births: preliminary data for 2014. Natl Vital Stat Rep. 2015;64(6):1–19.
61. Health AIo, Welfare. Australia's mothers and babies. Canberra: AIHW; 2021.
62. Wang Y, Tanbo T, Abyholm T, Henriksen T. The impact of advanced maternal age and parity on obstetric and perinatal outcomes in singleton gestations. Arch Gynecol Obstet. 2011;284(1):31–7.
63. Waldenstrom U, Aasheim V, Nilsen ABV, Rasmussen S, Pettersson HJ, Shytt E. Adverse pregnancy outcomes related to advanced maternal age compared with smoking and being overweight. Obstet Gynecol. 2014;123(1):104–12.
64. Gilliam M, Rosenberg D, Davis F. The likelihood of placenta previa with greater number of cesarean deliveries and higher parity. Obstet Gynecol. 2002;99(6):976–80.
65. National Center for Chronic Disease Prevention and Health Promotion DoRH. Assisted Reproductive Technology (ART) 2018 [updated April 20, 2021. https://www.cdc.gov/art/artdata/index.html.
66. Esh-Broder E, Ariel I, Abas-Bashir N, Bdolah Y, Celnikier DH. Placenta accreta is associated with IVF pregnancies: a retrospective chart review. BJOG. 2011;118(9):1084–9.

67. Kayem G, Seco A, Beucher G, Dupont C, Branger B, Crenn Hebert C, et al. Clinical profiles of placenta accreta spectrum: the PACCRETA population-based study. BJOG. 2021;128(10):1646–55.
68. Matsuzaki S, Nagase Y, Takiuchi T, Kakigano A, Mimura K, Lee M, et al. Antenatal diagnosis of placenta accreta spectrum after in vitro fertilization-embryo transfer: a systematic review and meta-analysis. Sci Rep. 2021;11(1):9205.
69. Kaser DJ, Melamed A, Bormann CL, Myers DE, Missmer SA, Walsh BW, et al. Cryopreserved embryo transfer is an independent risk factor for placenta accreta. Fertil Steril. 2015;103(5):1176–84 e2.
70. Saito K, Kuwahara A, Ishikawa T, Morisaki N, Miyado M, Miyado K, et al. Endometrial preparation methods for frozen-thawed embryo transfer are associated with altered risks of hypertensive disorders of pregnancy, placenta accreta, and gestational diabetes mellitus. Hum Reprod. 2019;34(8):1567–75.
71. Salmanian B, Fox KA, Arian SE, Erfani H, Clark SL, Aagaard KM, et al. In vitro fertilization as an independent risk factor for placenta accreta spectrum. Am J Obstet Gynecol. 2020;223(4):568. e1-e5
72. Jauniaux E, Alfirevic Z, Bhide AG, Belfort MA, Burton GJ, Collins SL, et al. Placenta praevia and placenta accreta: diagnosis and management: green-top guideline no. 27a. BJOG. 2019;126(1):e1–e48.
73. Baldwin HJ, Nippita TA, Torvaldsen S, Ibiebele I, Ford JB, Patterson JA. Outcomes of subsequent births after placenta accreta spectrum. Obstet Gynecol. 2020;136(4):745–55.
74. Sentilhes L, Kayem G, Ambroselli C, Provansal M, Fernandez H, Perrotin F, et al. Fertility and pregnancy outcomes following conservative treatment for placenta accreta. Hum Reprod. 2010;25(11):2803–10.
75. Chikazawa K, Imai K, Liangcheng W, Sasaki S, Horiuchi I, Kuwata T, et al. Detection of Asherman's syndrome after conservative management of placenta accreta: a case report. J Med Case Rep. 2018;12(1):344.
76. Brown AD, Hart JM, Modest AM, Hess PE, Abbas AM, Nieto-Calvache AJ, et al. Geographic variation in management of patients with placenta accreta spectrum: an international survey of experts (GPASS). Int J Gynaecol Obstet. 2021;
77. Lax A, Prince MR, Mennitt KW, Schwebach JR, Budorick NE. The value of specific MRI features in the evaluation of suspected placental invasion. Magn Reson Imaging. 2007;25(1):87–93.
78. Varghese B, Singh N, George RA, Gilvaz S. Magnetic resonance imaging of placenta accreta. Indian J Radiol Imaging. 2013;23(4):379–85.
79. Vinograd A, Wainstock T, Mazor M, Beer-Weisel R, Klaitman V, Dukler D, et al. Placenta accreta is an independent risk factor for late pre-term birth and perinatal mortality. J Matern Fetal Neonatal Med. 2015;28(12):1381–7.
80. Jauniaux E, Gronbeck L, Bunce C, Langhoff Roos J, Collins SL. Epidemiology of placenta previa accreta: a systematic review and meta-analysis. BMJ Open. 2019;9(11):e031193.
81. Wu S, Kocherginsky M, Hibbard JU. Abnormal placentation: twenty-year analysis. Am J Obstet Gynecol. 2005;192(5):1458–61.
82. Ornaghi S, Maraschini A, Donati S, Regional Obstetric Surveillance System Working G. Characteristics and outcomes of pregnant women with placenta accreta spectrum in Italy: a prospective population-based cohort study. PLoS One. 2021;16(6):e0252654.

Chapter 3
Pathogenesis of Placenta Accreta Spectrum

Erbil Karaman, Deniz Dirik, and Onur Karaaslan

Placenta accreta spectrum (PAS) is a placental abnormality that can cause severe maternal morbidity and mortality. PAS is abnormally invasive placental implantation due to decidua basalis defect. Abnormal adhesion of placenta to myometrium occurs through invasion of the myometrium by chorionic villi. Abnormal placental implantation or placental invasion is a potentially life-threatening complication in the third stage of delivery. It is primarily characterized by absence of decidua. Thus, chorionic villi are directly attached to myometrial fibers. Based on myometrial invasion depth of placental villi, PAS is classified into three categories, namely, placenta accreta, placenta increta, and placenta percreta. It is defined as placenta accreta if placental villi are localized adjacent to myometrium fibers in the absence of decidua, as placenta increta if placental villi invaded myometrium, and as placenta percreta if placenta invaded all layers of myometrium, uterine serosa, and even adjacent organs [1].

The placenta accreta is the mildest form among the three pathological conditions in which chorionic villi penetrate decidua. The placenta percreta is the most severe placental implantation anomaly and associated with serious maternal morbidity [2]. The abnormal adhesion may involve all cotyledons or a few cotyledons. Whole cotyledon or a part of single cotyledon may show adhesion. Clinically, abnormal placental invasions are termed as PAS in general since invasion could not be categorized clearly and villi can be at various invasion depths in same placental bed [3]. The diagnosis of PAS is made by histopathological examination. The

E. Karaman (✉)
Medical Faculty, Department of Obstetrics and Gynecology, Division of Gynecologic Oncology, Van Yuzuncu Yil University, Van, Turkey

D. Dirik · O. Karaaslan
Medical Faculty, Department of Obstetrics and Gynecology, Van Yuzuncu Yil University, Van, Turkey

S. A. Shazly, A. A. Nassr (eds.), *Placenta Accreta Spectrum*,
https://doi.org/10.1007/978-3-031-10347-6_3

histopathological diagnosis could not be established by placenta alone, and whole uterus or myometrial curettage may be needed for confirmation [4].

PAS has a wide clinical spectrum ranging from subclinical adhesion of myometrial fibers to placental basal layer to drastic clinical presentation of placenta percreta. Invasion depth of placental villi is the most important feature that determines severity of clinical presentation [1].

The mechanism leading to abnormal placentation is unclear although several risk factors have been established for PAS. Among mammalians, human placenta is almost disparate due to high invasiveness and complete embedment of conceptus into uterine decidua and endometrium [5]. In a healthy pregnancy, chorionic villi are implanted to spongious layer of decidua between gestational weeks 9 and 12. At proximal to placental basal layer, there is a cleavage line corresponding to demarcation line where chorion consisting of extracellular or fibrin material is separated from decidua. Interstitial trophoblasts invade myometrial tissue, while endovascular trophoblasts ensure remodeling of maternal spiral arteries, resulting in invasion of uterine wall by two groups of extravillous cytotrophoblasts [6]. As a result of such setup, placenta can separate from the cleavage line after delivery by myometrial contractions. This contributes postpartum hemostasis.

During implantation, cytotrophoblasts comprise branching villi and penetrate decidualized maternal stroma. These cells are nonproliferative and generally termed as extravillous trophoblast (EVT). The EVTs primarily transform into interstitial EVTs and endovascular EVTs, which advance to innermost layers of myometrium [5]. The outermost layer of myometrium is transformed into spiral arteries and includes basal arteries surrounding uterine glands [7]. The EVTs first appear around and within spiral arteries at placental area. These cells advance laterally and reach periphery of placenta. Invasion progressively advances toward periphery, while depth alterations are at maximum level in the central zone of placental bed [5]. In addition, human placenta is characterized by remodeling of spiral and basal arteries which occurs by loss of elastic lamina of vessels and response to several vasoactive compounds [7]. Both endovascular and interstitial EVT invasions are associated with physiological change of terminal part of uterine blood circulation. Thus, these cells play an important role in placentation by linking primitive placenta to uterus and modulating vascular changes in placental development. Total or partial loss of decidua is histological characteristic of PAS and can be clearly seen in implantation to uterine scar area [4]. In these cases, decidua is generally replaced by loose connective tissue, and placental villi are separated from myometrium fibers by a thin and irregular layer, namely, Nitabuch tissue, which may be absent in most cases. There may be local thinning in myometrium. Myometrium fibers may show degenerative changes with increased deposits of fibrous tissues and inflammatory cell infiltration; however, invasive villi are general normal in morphological manner [4]. The mechanism underlying abnormal implantation is inability to deep penetration of trophoblasts from defective decidua basalis in scarred inferior uterine segment. The major risk factors identified for PAS are placenta previa and previous history of cesarean section (C/S). The risk is increased by increasing number of previous C/S. Other risk factors include myometrial trauma, dilatation and curettage, maternal age, smoking, grand-multiparity, and recurrent fetal losses [2]. Theoretically, additional predisposing factors causing PAS such as endometritis, manual placenta removal, and other uterine anomalies can be associated with underdeveloped decidua. In all cases, normal superficial line over decidua basalis is disrupted, and complete placental removal does not occur after delivery.

A number of theories have been proposed to explain abnormal placentation in PAS. Former hypothesis was over-invasion to myometrium due to primary defect in trophoblast function [4]. Another hypothesis is that decidua basalis defect resulting from impaired normal decidualization at uterine scar area leads to abnormal depth of trophoblast invasion [4]. Some authors also proposed that local hypoxia secondary to abnormal vascularization during postoperative scarring process leads to both impaired decidualization and excessive trophoblast invasion [8]. It is known that there is history of cesarean section, curettage, and/or myomectomy in 80% of patients with PAS [4]. The increasing incidence of placenta previa due to previous C/S procedures supports scar formation at lower uterine segment and biological dysfunction of endometrium [1, 9–11]. Abnormal placentation may occur in localized defective areas resulting from interventions in uterine cavity such as cesarean, uterine curettage, and myomectomy, which may lead to placental invasion anomaly. However, in rare instances, uterine abnormalities such as bicornuate uterus, adenomyosis, or submucosal fibroids can be associated with microscopic endometrial defects by impairing normal endometrial functions, allowing abnormal placental implantation [12]. This may explain PAS rarely seen in primigravida women with no history of uterine surgery.

In a healthy pregnancy, primary invasive trophoblastic cell type in mononuclear cells forms multinucleated giant cells with low invasion potential. The giant cells are known as terminal step in the differentiation of extravillous trophoblasts. Smaller number of giant cells is seen in placental area of myometrium in specimens obtained from cases with PAS. This suggests that there is an abnormality in trophoblast itself or other regulatory factors. In addition, myometrial spiral arterioles with trophoblastic giant cell infiltration were seen in almost one-half of PAS cases, while such changes were seen in only 20% of patients with normal implantation [1, 13].

In PAS, EVTs localized at maternoplacental distance differ from giant syncytiotrophoblasts in normal placenta [14]. In particular, it was found that many EVTs showed cytotrophoblastic differences in pathology studies. The differences are generally hypertrophic and appear as thickening in implantation area by an increasing number. In addition to the increasing numbers of PAS, association of EVT with it is more common [14]. However, there is no difference in proliferative index apoptosis rate of trophoblastic cells localized in the middle of implantation area between normal implanted placenta and PAS [14].

It is known that endometrial glands are vital for fetal nutrition from implantation to intervillous circulation [15, 16]. The development of human fetoplacental unit occurs in a medium with low oxygen content via histiotrophic nutrition (at cellular level) from endometrial glands during most time in the first trimester. Through the end of the first trimester, intrauterine environment shows a radical change by the start of maternal arterial intervillous circulation and transition to hemotrophic nutrition [16, 17]. By elevation in intraplacental oxygen concentration, widespread villous remodeling is started in placental tissues [18]. The implantation relies on relationship between transformed endometrial cells and trophectoderm of blastocyst. It was shown that many regulatory molecules are involved in normal decidualization, control of trophoblastic adhesion, invasion, and governing penetration [19]. In general, it is known that there is a need for vascular endothelial growth factor (VEGF), placental growth factor (PIGF), and soluble Flt-1 (sFlt-1) release as well as equilibrium between these substances and oxygenation that regulates their release [20, 21]. Hypoxia triggers EVT proliferation and VEGF and mRNA expression, while normal oxygen has inhibitory effect. Interstitial EVT proteases degrade extracellular matrix and induce cell migration. Decidua prevents excessive spread of EVTS via tissue inhibitors such as matrix metalloproteinases and activity of many coagulation proteases [22]. In PAS, syncytiotrophoblast VEGF and epidermal growth factor receptor (EGFR) expressions are increased; it is known that PAS develops due to abnormal expression growth-, angiogenesis-, and invasion-related factors in trophoblastic population [23]. It was reported that lower maternal level of free VEGF is effective in transforming interstitial EVTS into metastatic phenotype in placenta previa, leading to excessive myometrial invasion of EVTs [8]. It was shown that the number of multinucleated giant cells was decreased in the decidua basalis of women with placenta previa or placenta accreta [8]. Syncytial fusion to multinucleated giant cells is another mechanism in the absence of invasion phenotype in EVTS. It is thought that VEGF released from multinucleated giant cells is one of the signals that coordinate and promote vascularization in decidua and placenta during placental implantation [16]. These findings support that VEGF play an important role in pathological programming of EVT motility and invasiveness [8].

In fallopian tubes, early placental development and placentation are similar to those occurring in uterus. Tubal placentation is generally membranous due to insufficient blood flow. The most common histological finding related to tubal pregnancy is chronic change of tubal endoepithelium. The role of chronic change in tubal implantation is similar to mechanism underlying implantation to C/S scar at lower uterine segment and subsequent placenta previa [16, 24]. None of trophoblastic changes seen in PAS was observed following tubal implantation, indicating that tubal process is less dependent to trophoblastic tissue function. In addition, it also supports that morphological changes seen in PAS EVTs are environmental and result of prolonged interaction between highly vascularized profound endometrium and EVTS. It was shown that complete loss of myometrium together with defective uterine scar can lead placenta percreta which may lead uterine rupture in the first half of gestation [25]. Although this is a rare complication, mechanism underlying placenta percreta-related uterine rupture is similar to tubal rupture in ectopic placentation. These findings emphasize the role of superficial endometrium in the modulation of uterine placentation. Superficial endometrium is important in dysfunctional decidualization secondary to excessive trophoblastic invasion. The leukocyte recruitment into endometrium during secretory phase following C/S supports the assumption that abnormal decidualization and trophoblastic changes in placental bed are secondary to uterine scar in PAS [26]. A human embryo develops in a relatively hypoxic environment and data from in vitro studies showed that oxygenation regulates placental development by deciding whether cytotrophoblasts will proliferate or invade [21]. Embryos may prefer to implant in uterine scar regions due to less vascularization and lower oxygen pressure.

References

1. Khong TY. The pathology of placenta accreta, a worldwide epidemic. J Clin Pathol. 2008;61(12):1243–6.
2. Piñas Carrillo A, Chandraharan E. Placenta accreta spectrum: risk factors, diagnosis and management with special reference to the Triple P procedure. Womens Health (Lond). 2019;15:1745506519878081.
3. Bartels HC, Postle JD, Downey P, Brennan DJ. Placenta accreta spectrum: a review of pathology, molecular biology, and biomarkers. Dis Markers. 2018;2018:1507674.
4. Baergen R. Placental pathology, an issue of surgical pathology clinics, E-book. Elsevier Health Sciences; 2013.
5. Burton GJ, Kaufmann P, Huppertz B. Anatomy and genesis of the placenta. Knobil and Neill's physiology of reproduction. 2006;1:189–244.
6. Pijnenborg R. The human decidua as a passage-way for trophoblast invasion: a review. Placenta. 1998;19:229–41.
7. Burton GJ, Woods AW, Jauniaux E, Kingdom JC. Rheological and physiological consequences of conversion of the maternal spiral arteries for uteroplacental blood flow during human pregnancy. Placenta. 2009;30(6):473–82.
8. Wehrum MJ, Buhimschi IA, Salafia C, Thung S, Bahtiyar MO, Werner EF, et al. Accreta complicating complete placenta previa is characterized by reduced systemic levels of vascular endothelial growth factor and by epithelial-to-mesenchymal transition of the invasive trophoblast. Am J Obstet Gynecol. 2011;204(5):411. e1-.e11
9. Hull AD, Moore TR. Multiple repeat cesareans and the threat of placenta accreta: incidence, diagnosis, management. Clin Perinatol. 2011;38(2):285–96.
10. Jauniaux E, Jurkovic D. Placenta accreta: pathogenesis of a 20th century iatrogenic uterine disease. Placenta. 2012;33(4):244–51.
11. Tantbirojn P, Crum CP, Parast MM. Pathophysiology of placenta creta: the role of decidua and extravillous trophoblast. Placenta. 2008;29(7):639–45.
12. Jauniaux E, Collins S, Burton GJ. Placenta accreta spectrum: pathophysiology and evidence-based anatomy for prenatal ultrasound imaging. Am J Obstet Gynecol. 2018;218(1):75–87.
13. Khong TY, De Wolf F, Robertson WB, Brosens I. Inadequate maternal vascular response to placentation in pregnancies complicated by pre-eclampsia and by small-for-gestational age infants. Br J Obstet Gynaecol. 1986;93(10):1049–59.
14. Kim KR, Jun SY, Kim JY, Ro JY. Implantation site intermediate trophoblasts in placenta cretas. Mod Pathol. 2004;17(12):1483–90.
15. Hempstock J, Cindrova-Davies T, Jauniaux E, Burton GJ. Endometrial glands as a source of nutrients, growth factors and cytokines during the first trimester of human pregnancy: a morphological and immunohistochemical study. Reprod Biol Endocrinol. 2004;2:58.
16. Moser G, Windsperger K, Pollheimer J, de Sousa Lopes SC, Huppertz B. Human trophoblast invasion: new and unexpected routes and functions. Histochem Cell Biol. 2018;150(4):361–70.
17. Burton GJ, Jauniaux E, Watson AL. Maternal arterial connections to the placental intervillous space during the first trimester of human pregnancy: the Boyd collection revisited. Am J Obstet Gynecol. 1999;181(3):718–24.
18. Jauniaux E, Poston L, Burton GJ. Placental-related diseases of pregnancy: involvement of oxidative stress and implications in human evolution. Hum Reprod Update. 2006;12(6):747–55.

19. Knöfler M. Critical growth factors and signalling pathways controlling human trophoblast invasion. Int J Dev Biol. 2010;54(2–3):269–80.
20. Ahmed A, Dunk C, Ahmad S, Khaliq A. Regulation of placental vascular endothelial growth factor (VEGF) and placenta growth factor (PIGF) and soluble Flt-1 by oxygen—a review. Placenta. 2000;21(Suppl A):S16-24.
21. Chang CW, Wakeland AK, Parast MM. Trophoblast lineage specification, differentiation and their regulation by oxygen tension. J Endocrinol. 2018;236(1):R43-r56.
22. Fluhr H, Krenzer S, Zygmunt M. Different regulation of tissue inhibitors of metalloproteinases-1, −2 and −3 in human endometrial stromal cells during decidualization in vitro. Reprod Med Biol. 2008;7(4):169–75.
23. Tseng JJ, Chou MM. Differential expression of growth-, angiogenesis- and invasion-related factors in the development of placenta accreta. Taiwan J Obstet Gynecol. 2006;45(2):100–6.
24. Hammer A. Immunological regulation of trophoblast invasion. J Reprod Immunol. 2011;90(1):21–8.
25. Jang DG, Lee GS, Yoon JH, Lee SJ. Placenta percreta-induced uterine rupture diagnosed by laparoscopy in the first trimester. Int J Med Sci. 2011;8(5):424–7.
26. Ben-Nagi J, Walker A, Jurkovic D, Yazbek J, Aplin JD. Effect of cesarean delivery on the endometrium. Int J Gynaecol Obstet. 2009;106(1):30–4.

Chapter 4
Anatomy of Placenta Accreta Spectrum

José M. Palacios-Jaraquemada, Nicolás Basanta, Álbaro Nieto-Calvache, and Rozi Aditya Aryananda

General Overview

Placenta accreta spectrum (PAS) is a challenging disease, closely associated with the increased number of cesarean sections worldwide [1]. In approximately 80% of the cases, PAS is about the posterior upper bladder. Still, the vascular anatomy and access could change for other locations, which implies advanced management of vascular anatomy and the pelvic fascia [2], due to the development of the newly formed vessels and a different degree of organ adhesion. In addition, prenatal studies habitually provide critical information to plan a surgery, but multiple biases [3] could affect studies. Consequently, not all prenatal evaluation is enough to know all invasion features.

Therefore, surgical staging is needed to manage all possible complications. During exploration, atraumatic maneuvers are essential. For this reason, knowledge of coalescence fascia [4] and pelvis spaces is strongly recommendable. Some invasion areas are highly complex by an affluent anastomotic net; by the proximity of vascular elements, narrow or deep access; or by a combination of all of these [5].

J. M. Palacios-Jaraquemada (✉)
CEMIC University Hospital and 1° Anatomy Chair, School of Medicine, University of Buenos Aires, Buenos Aires, Argentina

Universitas Airlangga, Surabaya, Indonesia

N. Basanta
Fernández Hospital and School of Medicine, 1° Anatomy Chair, University of Buenos Aires, Buenos Aires, Argentina

Á. Nieto-Calvache
Placenta Accreta Spectrum Clinic, Fundación Valle del Lili, Cali, Colombia

R. A. Aryananda
Dr. Soetomo Academic General Hospital, Universitas Airlangga, Surabaya, Indonesia

S. A. Shazly, A. A. Nassr (eds.), *Placenta Accreta Spectrum*, https://doi.org/10.1007/978-3-031-10347-6_4

The spatial location of components is essential to create a 3D conceptual representation before access [6]. Pelvic fascia management is not always part of the formal training of OBGYN; therefore, probably the best way to acquire skill managing [7] is guided teaching in unembalmed corpses.

Pelvic Spaces or Areas

Pelvic spaces are specific zones enclosed by two independent fasciae and filled with areolar connective tissue [8]. These areas could be exposed by dividing two independent fasciae along their cleavage plane, avascular and filled with fat or loose areolar connective tissues. This fact allows dissecting sheets and identifying elements without bleeding [9]. In addition, the wide opening of the pelvic para spaces allows the accurate identification and mobilization of structures. The anatomic demonstration is that pelvic spaces provide optimal conditions for conservative or resective procedures (Fig. 4.1).

Vesicouterine Space (VUS)

This space is handled for cesarean section, cesarean hysterectomy, or laparoscopic, robotic, or open laparotomy in obstetrics and gynecologic procedures [10]. The opening of the vesicovaginal space exposes the lower segment, the cervix, and the

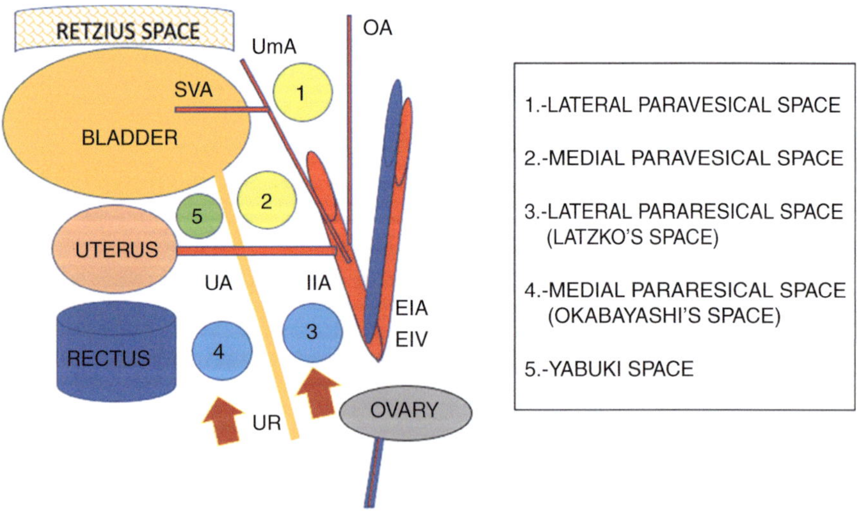

Fig. 4.1 Female pelvic spaces. *UmA* umbilical artery, *OA* obturator artery, *SVA* superior vesical artery, *UA* uterine artery, *IIA* iliac internal artery, *EIA* external iliac artery, *EIV* external iliac vein, *UR* ureter

upper vagina. The vesicouterine pouch bends the peritoneum over the uterus and the bladder, creating a recess nearer to the anterior vaginal fornix. The vesicouterine sac is attached to the uterus, preventing the falling of the bladder beyond the uterus. In patients with prior cesarean deliveries, it is possible to see adhesions in this space, increasing the risk of bladder injury [11]. Dissection of the vesicouterine space [12] is particularly useful to perform a ligature of newly formed vessels in PAS (Fig. 4.2).

Paracervical Space

A parallel and lateral space adjacent to the cervix and the bladder could be created by blunt dissection of the anterior leaf of the broad ligament [13]. This medial and inferior dissection lateral to the cervix is best to avoid injury to adjacent structures in the pelvic sidewall and allows identifying the vesicovaginal and vesicocervical ligament. This space allows for the lateral and inferior displacement of the ureter; maneuvers may diminish ureter injury by pushing it away by dissection planes during resective procedures, like the hysterectomy. Continued traction is maintained by keeping the medial aspect of the anterior leaf of the broad ligament intact [8]. The inverse vesicouterine fold dissection can be performed from this space. The vesicovaginal and vesicocervical area is developed from an unscarred plane [14]. This will safely separate the lowest portion of the bladder from the vagina, cervix, and uterus. Like the technique performed during a vaginal hysterectomy, this inverse motion of developing the bladder flap avoids erroneous and blind dissection through the vesicouterine adhesions.

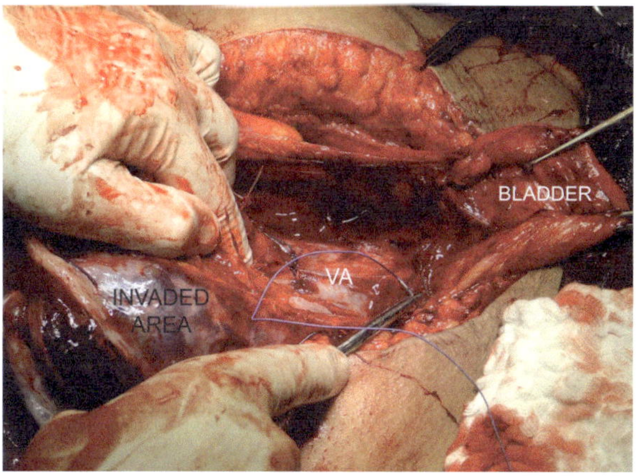

Fig. 4.2 Vesicouterine space (intraoperative). The vesicouterine space was wide open, and the needle ligates the colpouterine vessels, which runs inside of muscular vaginal layer. *VA*, vagina

Prevesical Space

The Retzius or prevesical space [15] is located between the pubis and the bladder, and it is filled by fat tissue (Fig. 4.3). It has complex communications with the adjacent pelvic extraperitoneal areas, rectus sheath, and retroperitoneum.

Several blood vessels are situated below pubis symphysis and laterally in the paravaginal space. There is an extensive plexus of veins, well-known as Santorini, and surgeons must be aware of their location [16]. The Santorini veins drain into the internal iliac vein. The dorsal vein of the clitoris runs caudally to the pubic symphysis and empties into the plexus of Santorini. The Retzius space is rarely affected in PAS. Still, sometimes, anterior invasion is attached to the anterior abdominal wall [17], and dissection of prevesical space is an excellent point to start a dissection to separate tissues from the rectus sheet. Notice that during anterior rectus muscle involvement, it needed to control the upper and the lower vascular pedicle (internal mammary artery and epigastric artery).

Paravesical Space

The paravesical space is covered by the peritoneum of the anterior leaf of the broad ligament (Fig. 4.3). Its floor is the iliococcygeus muscle and pubocervical fascia inserted into the arcus tendineus fascia pelvis [18]. The paravesical spaces lateral to the bladder communicate via the retropubic area in front of the bladder [18]. Paravesical space contains the umbilical artery, superior vesical artery, the obturator neurovascular bundle, lymphatic tissue, and some anastomotic vessels like the anastomosis between the obturator and epigastric artery—*corona mortis* [19]. The obliterated umbilical artery and prevesical umbilical fascia divide this space into lateral paravesical and medial paravesical space [20].

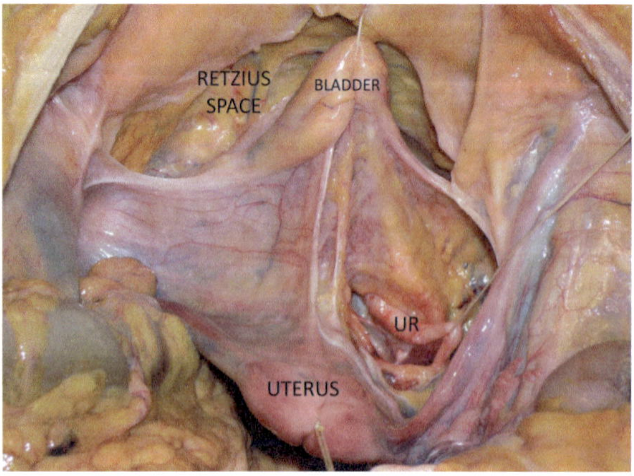

Fig. 4.3 Unembalmed corpse: superior viewing of the Retzius and paravesical space with the ureter

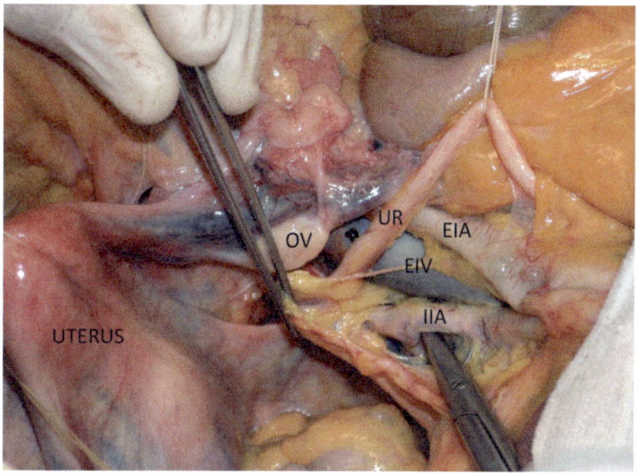

Fig. 4.4 Unembalmed corpse: right viewing of the pararectal space and the iliac vessels. The posterior peritoneum was opened 2 cm inside of the infundibulopelvic ligament. *OV* ovary, *UR* ureter, *EIA* external iliac artery, *EIV* external iliac vein, *IIA*, internal iliac artery

Pararectal Space

The pararectal space is in the posterior leaf of the broad ligament when the peritoneum is incised lateral to the infundibulopelvic ligament; the ureter is the first structure that appears after a minor dissection [21]. The ureter, or according to others, the hypogastric nerve, divides the pararectal space [8] into medial (Okabayashi's area) and lateral (Latzko's area) pararectal spaces (Fig. 4.4).

Parametrial Space

The parametrial space is located between the leaves of the broad ligament [22]. It is formed by the fibrous and fatty connective tissue that surrounds the uterus. It is bordered laterally by the internal iliac vessels, medially by the uterus, superiorly by the peritoneum, and inferiorly by the ureter [23]. This tissue contains the uterine artery and the superficial uterine vein (Fig. 4.5). Its access is invaluable to identify and characterize a placenta invasion of the parametrium. The parametrial space could be divided into the upper and lower area. The upper area involves the space above the peritoneal reflection in the pelvic floor and the lower one below them. The access is granted after cutting the anterior sheet of the broad ligament by the inner side of the round ligament [24]. Then an index finger enters between both sheets of the broad ligaments to separate the fat tissue and the ureter against the pelvic wall. Blunt dissection allows seeing the tissues until the pelvic floor. If cutting continues from the inner side of the round ligament, it is possible to enter the retrovesical space and connect both sides behind the bladder [25]. The lower parametrium is the most complicated area because it includes the ureter, fat tissue, lymphatics [18], and some anastomotic vessels in a narrow and deep space.

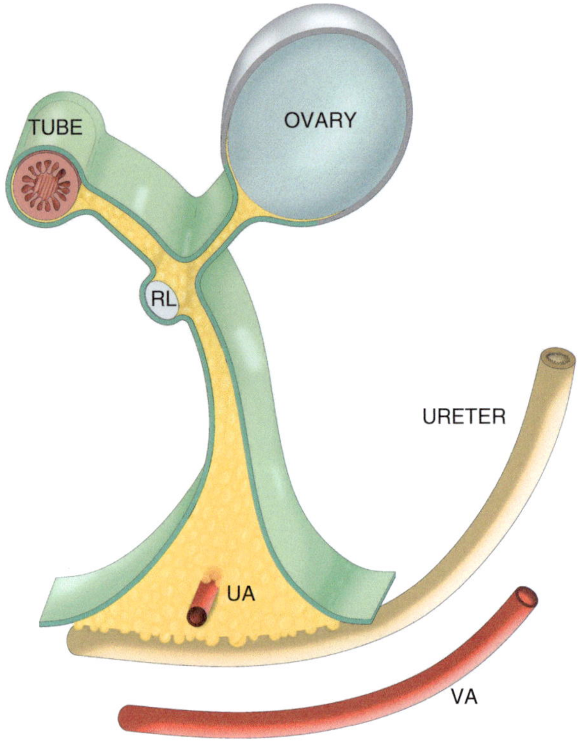

Fig. 4.5 Schematic sagittal cut of the broad ligament showing the parametrial space. *UA* uterine artery, *VA* vaginal artery from an internal pudendal artery, *RL* round ligament

Vascular Anatomy

Pelvic vessels mainly originate from internal iliac vessels, but this system receives blood from aortic, iliac external, and femoral components from anastomotic channels [26]. This network is continuously open to working immediately [27], without delay.

Proximal Vascular Control

The concept of proximal control includes the vessel and the anastomotic component. The most common cause of hemostasis failure is not to consider the blood flow by anastomotic or alternative pathways.

Uterine Vascular Areas

For many years, the medical community considered that the uterine blood supply was formed for the uterine arteries (80% of blood flow) and the ovary arteries (20% of blood flow). For decades it was considered that, after the occlusion of the uterine arteries, the upper pedicle, ovary arteries, and the round ligament artery replaced the uterine blood flow [28] after the vascular studies performed before the uterine transplantation proved that it was not valid. In 2006 [29], an anatomic study rediscovered a lower uterine anastomotic system that replaces the blood flow after ligature or embolization of uterine arteries. The lower system depends on the internal pudendal artery below the peritoneal reflection. Accordingly, the internal female reproductive organs are divided perpendicular to the posterior bladder wall. S1 area is irrigated by the uterine and ovary arteries and involves the uterine body. S2 area is irrigated by pelvisubperitoneal pedicles, such as the internal pudendal artery and their branches, and involves the lower uterine segment, the cervix, and the upper vagina. Understanding this division is essential to choose the most appropriate proximal vascular control [30].

In cases of PAS, the placenta needs an additional blood supply that is taken from surrounding vessels. Therefore, the anatomy of these vessels is key to planning an approach and optimal vascular control [31]. The embryological study of the pelvic vessels showed that a primary vascular sprout is dividing during organ development, but some connections among organs remain microscopically. In the presence of growth or vascular factors, these networks enlarge and create the "*newly-formed* vessels," and this process is called angiogenesis, which is defined as a physiological process through which new blood vessels form from preexisting vessels [32] built in the earlier stage of vasculogenesis. Angiogenesis continues the growth of the microscopical vasculature by methods of sprouting and splitting [33]. These vessels do not present a typical muscular, vascular layer; the muscular layer is underdeveloped concerning the systemic arteries.

Anterior Placenta Invasion

Posterior Upper Bladder

Approximately 80% of PAS cases concern the posterior upper bladder [24], which coincides with the most common hysterotomy level. Vessel connection among the placenta, uterus, and bladder is below the peritoneal reflection after opening a vesicouterine space between the round ligaments. The anterior sheet of the broad ligament is cut inside of obliterated umbilical artery bilaterally. An index finger passes through behind the bladder to isolate vessels by a vessel of a small group of them. In adherence to the posterior upper bladder, a finger passes through the cervix and the trigon. Then, a finger is pulled up to identify fibrous adherence and vessels [11]. When the pelvic fascia is not open, some surgeons push down the tissues behind the bladder, but it is highly possible to produce a vessel or a posterior bladder rupture. Connections between uterine or placenta vessels (from a uterine artery) and the vesical arteries are common in the upper posterior bladder [34]. Vascular components from the uterus and the placenta cross the vesicouterine space (Fig. 4.6); when the bladder is pulled up and down, the vesicouterine area opens, isolating and ligature of the newly formed vessels is more comfortable and safer.

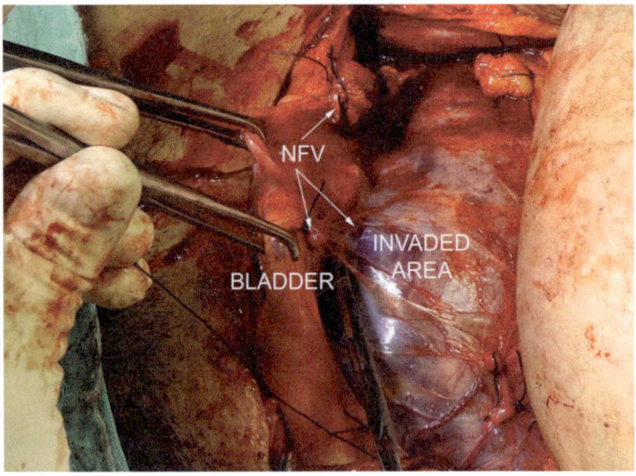

Fig. 4.6 Intraoperative view of ligature newly formed vessels in the vesicouterine space. *NFV*, newly formed vessels

Posterior Lower Bladder

Placenta invasion in the posterior lower bladder is not expected [35]. It is particularly blood supply and the collateral anastomotic system could be a nightmare even for a highly trained specialist. This area is deep and narrow, so it is needed excellent exposure and vascular image representation to avoid any unexpected or massive bleeding. This area is located among the trigon and the anterior cervix and the upper vagina and receives vessels from both vesical arteries (upper and lower), the upper vaginal artery (uterine artery), the middle vaginal artery (internal iliac artery), the lower vaginal artery (internal pudendal artery), and the cervical artery [36]. These vessels are part of a lower anastomotic ring that increases its volume and thickness in placenta invasion. In cases of posterior lower placenta invasion, it is possible to see two scenarios: (1) multiple vessels with a dissection plane between trigon and cervix and (2) many vessels and dense fibrosis between trigon and cervix. Deep dissection is possible to perform a ligature of the newly formed vessels, but the presence of fibrosis makes impossible a safe dissection; consequently, if it produces some injuries, it could end in massive and uncontrollable bleeding. Embolization in these circumstances is almost impossible due to the multiple vascular anastomotic channels. Pelvic packing is also inefficient because blood loss goes through to the retroperitoneum. Therefore, many PAS specialists avoid damage to the anastomotic ring (Fig. 4.7) by performing a subtotal hysterectomy.

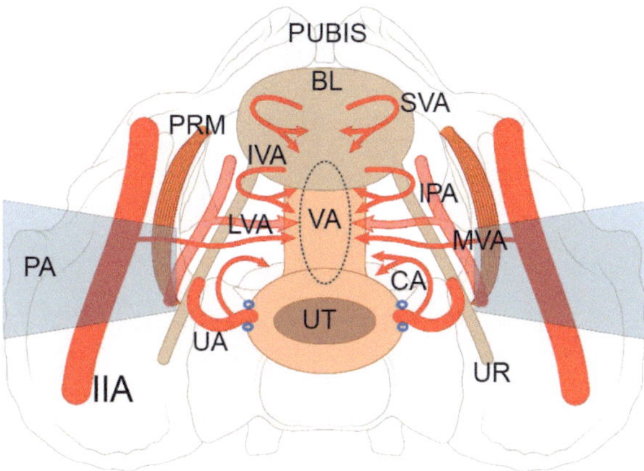

Fig. 4.7 Scheme of lower anastomotic ring. *BL* bladder, *SVA* superior vesical artery, *IVA* inferior vesical artery, *VA* vagina, *LVA* lower vaginal artery, *IPA* internal pudendal artery, *MVA* middle vaginal artery, *IIA* internal iliac artery, *UA* uterine artery, *CA* cervical artery, *UR* ureter, *UT* uterus

Lateral Invasion: The Parametrium

The parametrial invasion, especially the infraperitoneal area, is challenging to solve. Life-threatening bleeding is the leading cause of severe morbidity and mortality in PAS and is closely associated with cases of parametrial invasion. Anatomically, the parametrium is in the base of the broad ligament that includes the uterine artery, the ureter, lymph nodes, vessels, and fat tissue. As it happens with other pelvisubperitoneal spaces, the parametrium is widely connected to the retroperitoneum. Therefore, blood loss couldn't be evident in the pelvis, even with large volumes. In the absence of a TC, clinical suspicion and acidosis markers are our best options to detect hidden bleeding in the early stages. Diagnosis during surgical staging is mandatory after opening a space between twofold of the broad ligaments (Fig. 4.8); a Doyen or similar retractor is placed to separate virtual space. At this moment, we can find the following: (1) no placental tissue; (2) placental tissue covered by serosae, like lateral dehiscence; and (3) placental tissue and evident newly formed vessels [24].

In parametrial placenta invasion, ureter identification is mandatory. The ureters descend into the pelvis posterior to the infundibulopelvic ligaments in the upper pelvis. After crossing the iliac vessels, the ureters travel more medially. In this area, the ureter is 2 centimeters inside the infundibulopelvic ligament; when the posterior peritoneum is cut, the ureter moves up; you must take the ureter carefully and sling with thick silk or another element. This is because the ureter is surrounded by small vessels. If some maneuvers are not appropriately made, these vessels could break and develop a small hematoma that hides the ureter. After primary identification, the dissection must be followed by the anteromedial side of the ureter since a lateral side receives the ureteral blood supply. When dissection reaches the broad ligament, it is necessary to create a tunnel to identify the ureter in the anterior parametrium. The ureter is surrounded by loose connective tissue, making it easy to create a ureteral canal. The following important landmark is the transverse cervical ligament in

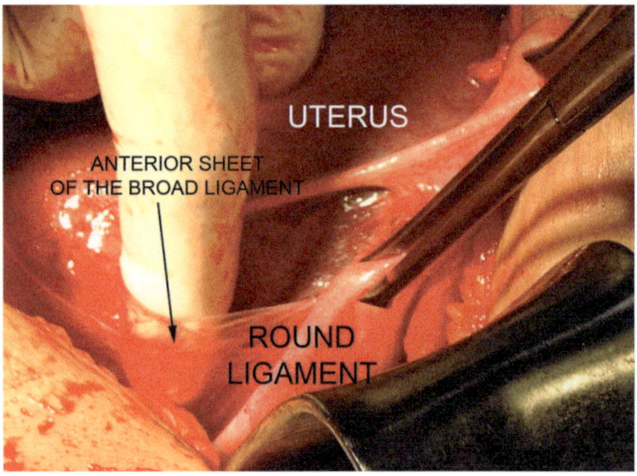

Fig. 4.8 Opening of parametrial space. Intraoperative

the lower pelvis. The ureters travel medially toward the bladder after passing under the transverse cervical ligament. Their insertion into the inferior aspect of the bladder is the third central location they should undergo identification intraoperatively [4]. In parametrial invasion, there are some problems, narrow space, newly formed vessels from the ureter, and branches of the internal iliac artery. In addition, part of the iliac branches are branches from the anterior division, but below peritoneal reflection, most vessels arose from the internal pudendal artery. This complex vascular net obliges to perform an upper vascular control, such as the infrarenal aorta.

Posterior Invasion

There is scarce information about the posterior invasion; although some authors comment on hemostasis problems in posterior placenta invasion, they do not provide details of possible problems and solutions. Placenta posterior invasion is associated with abortions, recurrent D&C, manual removal of the placenta, and large posterior myomectomies. The posterior uterine wall is thick, and significant damage is necessary to produce abnormal placentation. A superior third of the posterior wall receives blood supply from the uterine and ovary arteries, mesenteric arteries, or omentum [37]. The upper posterior uterus may also receive blood supply from the lumbar arteries [38]. In organ involvement, the newly formed pedicles originate from the organ that adheres to the posterior wall, large and small gut, and the omentum.

For this reason, proximal vascular control could be immediately below renal arteries to have control of the inferior mesenteric artery. A specific pedicle arises from the rectal artery in the lower and middle posterior areas. These tiny vessels enlarge significantly in cases of placenta invasion, and it could produce paradoxical severe bleeding even after aortic control (aortic division). We denominate this artery

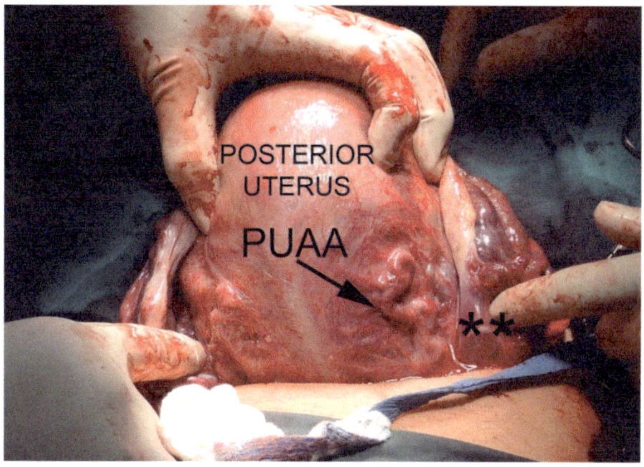

Fig. 4.9 Intraoperative view. Asterisk, right uterine pedicle; *PUAA* posterior uterine anastomotic artery

as the posterior uterine anastomotic artery (PUAA) (Fig. 4.9) that runs below the peritoneum and is easily visible after uterine exteriorization. It looks like a thick arterial vessel without a vein; it could be controlled with a simple ligature that includes 2 cm of the myometrium. Due to the reduced cases of posterior invasion and poor knowledge of this vessel, it is habitually an origin of massive bleeding. As with other uterine vessels, the PUAA is widely connected with the uterine and vaginal net and may cause unusual bleeding [39] by the uterus [40] or the vagina [39]. It is possible to see uterosacral ligaments in the low posterior and lateral uterus. They are another landmark to identify the ureter and the autonomic component of the pelvic viscera. When the posterior peritoneum is opening 2 cm lateral to the uterosacral ligament, the ureter is evident and easy for dissection or sling.

Uterine Blood Supply

Classically, the uterus has two pedicles, the uterine artery, which supplies 90% of the uterus, and the ovary arteries, providing 10% of the blood flow. Before 2006, it was described only as an upper anastomotic vessel, the round ligament artery, which arises from the epigastric artery. After this date, a lower extrauterine anastomotic system was described [29], which replaces a uterine blood flow after ligature or embolization of the uterine arteries. This system mainly depends on the internal pudendal branches, especially the lower vaginal artery. A perpendicular line that crosses the posterior bladder wall determines two uterine vascular areas. S1 involves the uterine body and the upper part of the uterine segment, and S2 affects the lower uterine segment, the cervix, and the upper vagina [41]. Apart from these areas, it is possible to recognize specific ones in the female reproductive system that determine specific vessels by topographic areas [42] and methods for proximal vascular control (Table 4.1). Due to most PAS cases about the posterior upper bladder (lower segment), vascular controls that affect only the uterine artery (like embolization or

Table 4.1 Female organs' blood supply

Sectors	S1	S2	S3	S4	S5
Location	Uterine body Upper uterine segment	Lower uterine segment Cervix and upper vagina	Middle and lower vagina	Upper posterior Uterus	Lower posterior uterus
Vessels	Uterine (IIA) and ovary artery (AO)	Cervical artery, upper vaginal artery (UA) Middle vaginal artery (IIA) Lower vaginal artery (IPA) Upper and lower vesical arteries	Lower vaginal artery (IPA)	Ovary and uterine artery Omental artery Superior and inferior mesenteric artery (AO) Round ligament artery (EA)	Ovary (AO) and uterine artery (IIA) Posterior uterine anastomotic artery
Proximal vascular control	Fallopian tube-uterine junction Uterine artery (horizontal) Iliac internal (CIA)	Compression suture over bleeding point Lower infrarenal aorta External or internal compression, sling, or balloon Common iliac artery (bilateral)	Compression suture over bleeding point Lower infrarenal aorta External or internal compression, sling, or balloon Bilateral balloon of common iliac artery (AO)	Rubber tube around the uterine body Fallopian tube-uterine junction	Upper infrarenal aorta External or internal compression, sling, or balloon

UA uterine artery, *AO* abdominal aorta, *IPA* internal pudendal artery, *CIA* common iliac artery, *IIA* iliac internal artery, *EA* epigastric artery

ligature) are not always efficient to avoid blood loss [43]. Something similar happens with internal iliac control because most of the branches in the lower segment, upper vagina, and posterior bladder originate from the posterior division of internal iliac arteries. This data is proved by randomized control trials and systematic review studies [44].

Anatomy Learning for Surgeons

Dissection allows the 3D conception of the subject matter and the interrelationships of anatomical structures. It also encourages the improvement of manual dexterity and an appreciation of a different anatomical variation, as seen between altered. There is a big difference in surgeons who had anatomical training or not. Although it is possible to perform a surgery moving and pushing tissues, there is an enormous difference when the surgeon finds the structures with anatomical knowledge or skills [45]. Anatomy is needed to be planned and implemented in postgraduate training to avoid an inevitable decline in surgical standards. Doctors interested in interventionalist careers [46] such as surgery need support in anatomy with direction from educators who have clinical experience. Complete training in human structure is core to operating training to warrant safety in practice in the surgical room, especially in hazardous procedures. Complete cadaver dissection constitutes the most effective training mode [47], especially for surgical specialties. Integrating human anatomy with other medical subjects is a helpful way of improving its retention and application.

Summary

Knowing the vascular and pelvic uterine relations allows us to plan a surgical approach to PAS. The opening of pelvic spaces is instrumental in dissecting specific areas and elements. Most vascular structures are infraperitoneal; consequently, the surgeon can perform precise vascular hemostasis after an accurate exposition. Topographic anatomy is needed for truthful management in some areas, such as the lower posterior bladder or the infraperitoneal parametrium. Finally, the expertise in pelvic and uterine pedicles is the best way to plan proper proximal vascular control. Although most cases of PAS are located about the upper posterior bladder, the precise management of all pelvic spaces and areas is necessary to control any possible variation. Anatomy skills are required to solve organ adhesions, understand the effectiveness of proximal vascular control, and manage unexpected situations.

Acknowledgments We sincerely thank Prof. Fabián Cabrera and Dr. Nicolás Rosasco for their help with the schemes.

References

1. To WW, Leung WC. Placenta previa and previous cesarean section. Int J Gynaecol Obstet. 1995;5(1):25–31. https://doi.org/10.1016/0020-7292(95)80004-v.
2. Cosma S, Ferraioli D, Mitidieri M, Ceccaroni M, Zola P, Micheletti L, Benedetto C. A simplified fascial model of pelvic anatomical surgery: going beyond parametrium-centered surgical anatomy. Anat Sci Int. 2021;96(1):20–9. https://doi.org/10.1007/s12565-020-00553-z. Epub 2020 Jun 11. PMID: 32529339; PMCID: PMC7806572
3. Bowman ZS, Eller AG, Kennedy AM, Richards DS, Winter TC 3rd, Woodward PJ, Silver RM. Accuracy of ultrasound for the prediction of placenta accreta. Am J Obstet Gynecol. 2014;211(2):177.e1-7. https://doi.org/10.1016/j.ajog.2014.03.029. Epub 2014 Mar 14
4. McEvoy A, Tetrokalashvili M. Anatomy, abdomen and pelvis, female pelvic cavity. [updated 2021 Jul 26]. In: StatPearls [internet]. Treasure Island, FL: StatPearls Publishing; 2021. https://www.ncbi.nlm.nih.gov/books/NBK538435/.

5. Lin CC, Adamczyk CJ, Montag AG, Zelop CM, Snow JC. Placenta previa percreta involving the left broad ligament and cervix. A case reports. J Reprod Med. 1998;43(9):839–43.
6. Flaxman TE, Cooke CM, Miguel OX, Sheikh AM, Singh SS. A review and guide to creating patient-specific 3D printed anatomical models from MRI for benign gynecologic surgery. 3D Print Med. 2021;7:17. https://doi.org/10.1186/s41205-021-00107-7.
7. Gilbody J, Prasthofer AW, Ho K, Costa ML. The use and effectiveness of cadaveric workshops in higher surgical training: a systematic review. Ann R Coll Surg Engl. 2011;93(5):347–52. https://doi.org/10.1308/147870811X582954. PMID: 21943455; PMCID: PMC3365449
8. Kostov S, Slavchev S, Dzhenkov D, Mitev D, Yordanov A. Avascular spaces of the female pelvis-clinical applications in obstetrics and gynecology. J Clin Med. 2020;9(5):1460. https://doi.org/10.3390/jcm9051460. PMID: 32414119; PMCID: PMC7291144
9. Ercoli A, Delmas V, Fanfani F, Gadonneix P, Ceccaroni M, Fagotti A, Mancuso S, Scambia G. Terminologia Anatomica versus unofficial descriptions and nomenclature of the fasciae and ligaments of the female pelvis: a dissection-based comparative study. Am J Obstet Gynecol. 2005;193(4):1565–73. https://doi.org/10.1016/j.ajog.2005.05.007.
10. Dubuisson JB., Dubuisson J., Puigventos J. Chapter: the vesicovaginal space. In: Laparoscopic anatomy of the pelvic floor. Cham: Springer; 2020. https://doi.org/10.1007/978-3-030-35498-5_12.
11. Rooney CM, Crawford AT, Vassallo BJ, Kleeman SD, Karram MM. Is previous cesarean section a risk for incidental cystotomy at the time of hysterectomy? A case-controlled study. Am J Obstet Gynecol. 2005;193(6):2041–4. https://doi.org/10.1016/j.ajog.2005.07.090.
12. Pelosi MA 3rd, Pelosi MA. Modified cesarean hysterectomy for placenta previa percreta with bladder invasion: retrovesical lower uterine segment bypass. Obstet Gynecol. 1999;93(5 Pt 2):830–3.
13. Sakuragi N, Kaneuchi M. Paracervical and paravaginal tissue dissection in the Okabayashi-Kobayashi radical hysterectomy and nerve-sparing technique. Int J Gynecol Cancer. 2021;31(1):145–6. https://doi.org/10.1136/ijgc-2020-002036. Free video.: https://ijgc.bmj.com/content/31/1/145
14. Nezhat C, Grace LA, Razavi GM, Mihailide C, Bamford H. Reverse vesicouterine fold dissection for laparoscopic hysterectomy after prior cesarean deliveries. Obstet Gynecol. 2016;128(3):629–33. https://doi.org/10.1097/AOG.0000000000001593.
15. Kim SW, Kim HC, Yang DM, Min GE. The prevesical space: anatomical review and pathological conditions. Clin Radiol. 2013;68(7):733–40. https://doi.org/10.1016/j.crad.2013.01.010. Epub 2013 Mar 7
16. Awad A, Alsaid B, Bessede T, Droupy S, Benoît G. Evolution in the concept of erection anatomy. Surg Radiol Anat. 2011;33(4):301–12. https://doi.org/10.1007/s00276-010-0707-4. Epub 2010 Aug 5
17. Abbas AM, Ali SEA, Michael A, Ali SS. Successful fertility-preserving management of a case of placenta percreta invading the urinary bladder and anterior abdominal wall: a case report. Middle East Fertil Soc J. 2018;23:77–80.
18. Lichtenegger W, Anderhuber F, Ralph G. 10 operative anatomy and technique of radical parametrial resection in the surgical treatment of cervical cancer. Baillieres Clin Obstet Gynaecol. 1998;2(4):841–56. https://doi.org/10.1016/s0950-3552(98)80012-6.
19. Cardoso GI, Chinelatto LA, Hojaij F, Akamatsu FE, Jacomo AL. Corona mortis: a systematic review of literature. Clinics (Sao Paulo). 2021;76:e2182. https://doi.org/10.6061/clinics/2021/e2182. PMID: 33886786; PMCID: PMC8024925
20. Yabuki Y, Sasaki H, Hatakeyama N, et al. Discrepancies between classic anatomy and modern gynecologic surgery on pelvic connective tissue structure: harmonization of those concepts by collaborative cadaver dissection. Am J Obstet Gynecol. 2005;193:7–15.
21. Dietrich CS 3rd, Gehrich A, Bakaya S. Surgical exposure and anatomy of the female pelvis. Surg Clin North Am. 2008;88(2):223–43., v. https://doi.org/10.1016/j.suc.2008.01.003.
22. Viswanathan AN, Dizon DS, Gien LT, Koh W-J. Chapter 58 - cervical cancer. In: Leonard L, Gunderson LL, Tepper JE, editors. Clinical radiation oncology (fourth edi-

tion). Elsevier; 2016. p. 1173–1202.e6. https://doi.org/10.1016/B978-0-323-24098-7.00058-7. ISBN 9780323240987 (https://www.sciencedirect.com/science/article/pii/B9780323240987000587).

23. Chopin N, Vieira M, Borghese B, Foulot H, Dousset B, Coste J, Mignon A, Fauconnier A, Chapron C. Operative management of deeply infiltrating endometriosis: results on pelvic pain symptoms according to a surgical classification. J Minim Invasive Gynecol. 2005;12(2):106–12. https://doi.org/10.1016/j.jmig.2005.01.015.
24. Palacios-Jaraquemada JM, Fiorillo A, Hamer J, Martínez M, Bruno C. Placenta accreta spectrum: a hysterectomy can be prevented in almost 80% of cases using a resective-reconstructive technique. J Matern Fetal Neonatal Med. 2020;26:1–8. https://doi.org/10.1080/14767058.2020.1716715. Epub ahead of print
25. Muallem MZ, Armbrust R, Neymeyer J, Miranda A, Muallem J. Nerve sparing radical hysterectomy: short-term oncologic, surgical, and functional outcomes. Cancers (Basel). 2020;12(2):483. https://doi.org/10.3390/cancers12020483. PMID: 32092946; PMCID: PMC7072686
26. Chait A, Moltz A, Nelson JH Jr. The collateral arterial circulation in the pelvis. An angiographic study. Am J Roentgenol Radium Therapy, Nucl Med. 1968;102(2):392–400. https://doi.org/10.2214/ajr.102.2.392.
27. Shrestha R, Shrestha S, Sitaula S, Basnet P. Anatomy of internal iliac artery and its ligation to control pelvic Hemorrhage. JNMA J Nepal Med Assoc. 2020;58(230):826–30. https://doi.org/10.31729/jnma.4958. PMID: 34504379; PMCID: PMC7654485
28. Worthington-Kirsch RL. Uterine artery embolization: state of the art. Semin Intervent Radiol. 2004;21(1):37–42. https://doi.org/10.1055/s-2004-831403. PMID: 21331107; PMCID: PMC3036203
29. Palacios Jaraquemada JM, García Mónaco R, Barbosa NE, Ferle L, Iriarte H, Conesa HA. Lower uterine blood supply: extrauterine anastomotic system and its application in surgical devascularization techniques. Acta Obstet Gynecol Scand. 2007;86(2):228–34. https://doi.org/10.1080/00016340601089875.
30. Palacios-Jaraquemada JM. Proximal vascular control in cases of abnormal placentation. Int J Obstet Anesth. 2011;20(3):266. https://doi.org/10.1016/j.ijoa.2011.01.002. Epub 2011 Jun 2
31. Ishibashi H, Miyamoto M, Iwahashi H, Matsuura H, Kakimoto S, Sakamoto T, Hada T, Takano M. Criteria for placenta accreta spectrum in the International Federation of Gynaecology and Obstetrics classification, and topographic invasion area are associated with massive hemorrhage in patients with placenta previa. Acta Obstet Gynecol Scand. 2021;100(6):1019–25. https://doi.org/10.1111/aogs.14143. Epub 2021 Mar 23
32. Nova Science. Angiogenesis insights from a systematic overview. New York: Nova Science; 2013. ISBN 978-1-62618-114-4
33. Flamme I, Frölich T, Risau W. Molecular mechanisms of vasculogenesis and embryonic angiogenesis. J Cell Physiol. 1997;173(2):206–10. https://doi.org/10.1002/(SICI)1097-4652(199711)173:2<206::AID-JCP22>3.0.CO;2-C.
34. Palacios Jaraquemada JM, Pesaresi M, Nassif JC, Hermosid S. Anterior placenta percreta: surgical approach, hemostasis and uterine repair. Acta Obstet Gynecol Scand. 2004;83(8):738–44. https://doi.org/10.1111/j.0001-6349.2004.00517.x.
35. Tinari S, Buca D, Cali G, Timor-Tritsch I, Palacios-Jaraquemada J, Rizzo G, Lucidi A, Di Mascio D, Liberati M, D'Antonio F. Risk factors, histopathology and diagnostic accuracy in posterior placenta accreta spectrum disorders: systematic review and meta-analysis. Ultrasound Obstet Gynecol. 2021;57(6):903–9. https://doi.org/10.1002/uog.22183.
36. González J, Albeniz LF, Ciancio G. Vascular problems of the pelvis. In: Lanzer P, editor. PanVascular Medicine. Berlin, Heidelberg: Springer; 2015. https://doi.org/10.1007/978-3-642-37078-6_152.
37. Anton K, Rosenblum NG, Teefey P, Dayaratna S, Gonsalves CF. The enlarged fibroid uterus: aberrant arterial supply via the omental artery. Cardiovasc Intervent Radiol. 2019;42(4):615–9. https://doi.org/10.1007/s00270-018-2087-9. Epub 2018 Oct 15

38. Pelage JP, Cazejust J, Pluot E, Le Dref O, Laurent A, Spies JB, Chagnon S, Lacombe P. Uterine fibroid vascularization and clinical relevance to uterine fibroid embolization. Radiographics. 2005;25(Suppl 1):S99-117. https://doi.org/10.1148/rg.25si055510.
39. Kim CH, Lee SJ, Jeon GS, Kang SH, Kim HC. Embolization of inferior mesenteric artery for intractable intrapelvic and vaginal bleeding after hysterectomy. J Minim Invasive Gynecol. 2016;23(7):1191–4. https://doi.org/10.1016/j.jmig.2016.07.013. Epub 2016 Jul 20
40. Shin SM, Yi KW, Chung HH. Postpartum uterine bleeding from the inferior mesenteric artery: case report and review of the literature. Gynecol Obstet Investig. 2015;80(1):60–3. https://doi.org/10.1159/000367598. Epub 2015 Feb 4
41. Uterovaginal Blood Supply: the S1 and S2 Segmental Concepts and their Clinical Relevance. Palacios-Jaraquemada JM, Karoshi M, Keith LG. Chapter 2. In: A Comprehensive Textbook of Postpartum Hemorrhage. An essential clinical reference for Effective Management Sapiens Publishing; 2012 2nd Revised edition.
42. Palacios-Jaraquemada JM. Efficacy of surgical techniques to control obstetric hemorrhage: analysis of 539 cases. Acta Obstet Gynecol Scand. 2011;90(9):1036–42. https://doi.org/10.1111/j.1600-0412.2011.01176.x. Epub 2011 Jun 14
43. Chou YJ, Cheng YF, Shen CC, Hsu TY, Chang SY, Kung FT. Failure of uterine arterial embolization: placenta accreta with profuse postpartum hemorrhage. Acta Obstet Gynecol Scand. 2004;83(7):688–90. https://doi.org/10.1046/j.0001-6349.2002.00002.x.
44. Liang D, Zhao H, Liu D, Lin Y. Internal iliac artery balloon occlusion in the management of placenta accreta: a systematic review and meta-analysis. Eur J Radiol. 2021;139:109711. https://doi.org/10.1016/j.ejrad.2021.109711. Epub 2021 Apr 20. PMID: 33910145
45. Ramsey S. Changing times, changing training: anatomy teaching in basic surgical training. Clin Anat. 2005;18(6):467–8. https://doi.org/10.1002/ca.20124.
46. Dangerfield PH. Medical science teaching needs stronger support from universities and a better career structure for anatomists. Clin Anat. 2005;18(6):468–9. https://doi.org/10.1002/ca.20123.
47. Ogeng'o JA. Anatomy training for surgeons: which way for the future? Ann Afr Surg. 2009;4:24–8.

Chapter 5
Classification of Placenta Accreta Spectrum

Rozi Aditya Aryananda and Grace Ariani

Introduction

Placenta accreta spectrum (PAS) is the term that describes the pathologic adherent of the placenta into the uterine wall without intervening decidua or basalis layer. The main mechanical risk factor of PAS is the cesarean section, curettage, or in vitro fertilization (IVF), and this is consistent with the possible cause of endometrial defect which leads to PAS in the next pregnancy [1, 2].

PAS is a heterogeneous condition associated with a high maternal morbidity and mortality rate, presenting unique challenges in diagnosis and management. It is caused by the lack of a standardized approach in reporting PAS cases for the ultrasound, clinical, and pathologic diagnosis [3]. PAS has many controversies and one of them is about the pre-, intra-, and postsurgical classification [4].

In the past, the diagnosis of placental implantation was only based on histopathology findings of cesarean hysterectomy, but several considerations related to uterine conservative surgery and the risk of bleeding during cesarean hysterectomy have made uterine conservative surgery an option in the management of PAS.

The traditional category only uses the terminologies placenta accreta, increta, and percreta based on histopathology and does not describe clinical criteria at the time of surgery. This traditional classification describes accreta invasion as placental villi adhering to the underlying myometrium, without an intervening layer of decidua, increta invasion as placental villi invading into the myometrial wall, and percreta invasion as placental villi invading through the full thickness of the

R. A. Aryananda (✉)
Maternal Fetal Medicine, Department of Obstetrics & Gynecology, Dr. Soetomo Academic General Hospital, Universitas Airlangga, Surabaya, Indonesia

G. Ariani
Department of Anatomical Pathology, Dr. Soetomo Academic General Hospital, Universitas Airlangga, Surabaya, Indonesia

S. A. Shazly, A. A. Nassr (eds.), *Placenta Accreta Spectrum*,
https://doi.org/10.1007/978-3-031-10347-6_5

myometrial wall to involve the uterine serosa [5, 6]. This traditional classification does not reflect the complexity of the surgery, and one placenta can have a different type of invasion and is highly dependent on sampling technique, so this classification has many weaknesses.

Clinicopathology Classification

There are two approaches used to describe the degree of PAS severity, clinical criteria during surgery and histopathological criteria. These two criteria have different approaches and important information, so they often cause controversy.

The clinical criteria for PAS used when placental tissue is present on the uterine surface can also lead to overdiagnosis because uterine dehiscence can have the same appearance as the PAS. Therefore, the clinical definition has to be the most important criterion for the definition of PAS [7].

The main histopathological criteria used to confirm the diagnosis of PAS were the absence of a decidual invasion and presence of placental invasion that penetrate the endometrial-myometrial layer, but this is a dilemmatic problem because the histopathological results are strongly influenced by surgical techniques and macroscopic sampling methods [8]. Different degrees of villous invasion have been described throughout the same placenta, with areas of accreta and percreta coexisting on the same specimen, further limiting the accuracy of microscopic diagnosis as it becomes dependent on the site of sampling.

One of the management of PAS is uterine resective-reconstructive surgery where the focal myometrial resection is applied in the abnormality of placental invasion [9]. The pathologist only obtained a focal myometrial resection with a placental attachment which was presumed to be the area of implantation of the placenta into the myometrium based on clinical findings during surgery. This conservative surgical technique presents a new challenge for the pathologist in the macroscopic examination of placental implantation, where it will be difficult to distinguish placental and uterine, especially on fresh tissue. Unfixation tissue is very soft and the myometrial sample is thin that it is sometimes difficult to find and distinguish, and for that a multidisciplinary team is needed. The existence of communication between the operator and the pathologist has an important role, where agreement on the provision of markers of the location of the placenta-uterine attachment during tissue delivery can help histopathological analysis. Histopathological diagnosis of PAS was confirmed by hysterectomy and uterine resective-reconstructive surgery, but histopathology diagnosis of PAS could not be confirmed if the sample received was only part of placental tissue which is taken during surgery or placental bed biopsy [3, 10].

Histopathological and clinical criteria controversies in PAS cause overdiagnosis of placental invasion disorders and bias to explain the epidemiology of PAS in the world. The International Federation of Gynaecology and Obstetrics (FIGO) made a consensus to bridge the clinical appearance and histopathological grading of PAS (Table 5.1) [1].

Table 5.1 The International Federation of Gynaecology and Obstetrics (FIGO) classification of placenta accreta spectrum

Grade	Clinical criteria	Histologic criteria
1 Abnormally adherent placenta (accreta) (Fig. 5.1)	At vaginal delivery: – No separation with synthetic oxytocin and gentle controlled cord traction. – Attempts at manual removal of the placenta results in heavy bleeding from the placenta implantation site requiring mechanical or surgical procedures. If laparotomy is required (including for cesarean delivery): – Same as above. – Macroscopically, the uterus shows no obvious distension over the placental bed (placental "bulge"), no placental tissue is seen invading through the surface of the uterus, and there is no or minimal neovascularity.	Microscopic examination of the placental bed samples from hysterectomy specimen shows extended areas of absent decidua between villous tissue and myometrium with placental villi attached directly to the superficial myometrium – The diagnosis cannot be made on just delivered placental tissue nor on random biopsies of the placental bed
2 Abnormally invasive placenta (increta) (Fig. 5.2)	At laparotomy: – Abnormal macroscopic findings over the placental bed: Bluish/ purple coloring, distension (placental "bulge"). – Significant amounts of hypervascularity (dense tangled bed of vessels or multiple vessels running parallel craniocaudially in the uterine serosa) – No placental tissue seen to be invading through the uterine serosa. – Gentle cord traction results in the uterus being pulled inward without separation of the placenta (so-called the dimple sign).	Hysterectomy specimen or partial myometrial resection of the increta area shows placental villi within the muscular fibers and sometimes in the lumen of the deep uterine vasculature (radial or arcuate arteries)
3 Abnormally invasive placenta (percreta)		

(continued)

Table 5.1 (continued)

Grade	Clinical criteria	Histologic criteria
3a Limited to the uterine serosa (Fig. 5.3)	At laparotomy: – Abnormal macroscopic findings on uterine serosal surface (as above) and placental tissue seen to be invading through the surface of the uterus. – No invasion into any other organ, including the posterior wall of the bladder (a clear surgical plane can be identified between the bladder and uterus).	Hysterectomy specimen showing villous tissue within or breaching the uterine serosa
3b with urinary bladder invasion (Fig. 5.4)	At laparotomy: – Placental villi are seen to be invading into the bladder but no other organs. – Clear surgical plane cannot be identified between the bladder and uterus.	Hysterectomy specimen showing villous tissue breaching the uterine serosa and invading the bladder wall tissue or urothelium
3c with invasion of other pelvic tissue or organ (Fig. 5.5)	At laparotomy: – Placental villi are seen to be invading into the broad ligament, vaginal wall, pelvic sidewall, or any other pelvic organ (with or without invasion of the bladder).	Hysterectomy specimen showing villous tissue breaching the uterine serosa and invading pelvic tissues/organs (with or without invasion of the bladder)

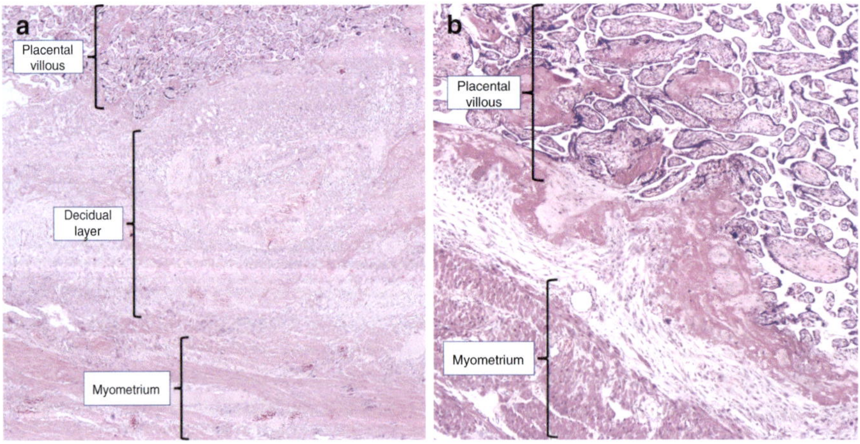

Fig. 5.1 (**a**) Area with normal implantation; decidual basalis layer is intact (orange arrow). H&E-stained section at ×10 magnification. (**b**) Placenta accreta; PAS grade 1. Loss of decidual layer in the area of placental implantation; placental villi attached directly to the superficial myometrium. H&E-stained section at ×100 magnification

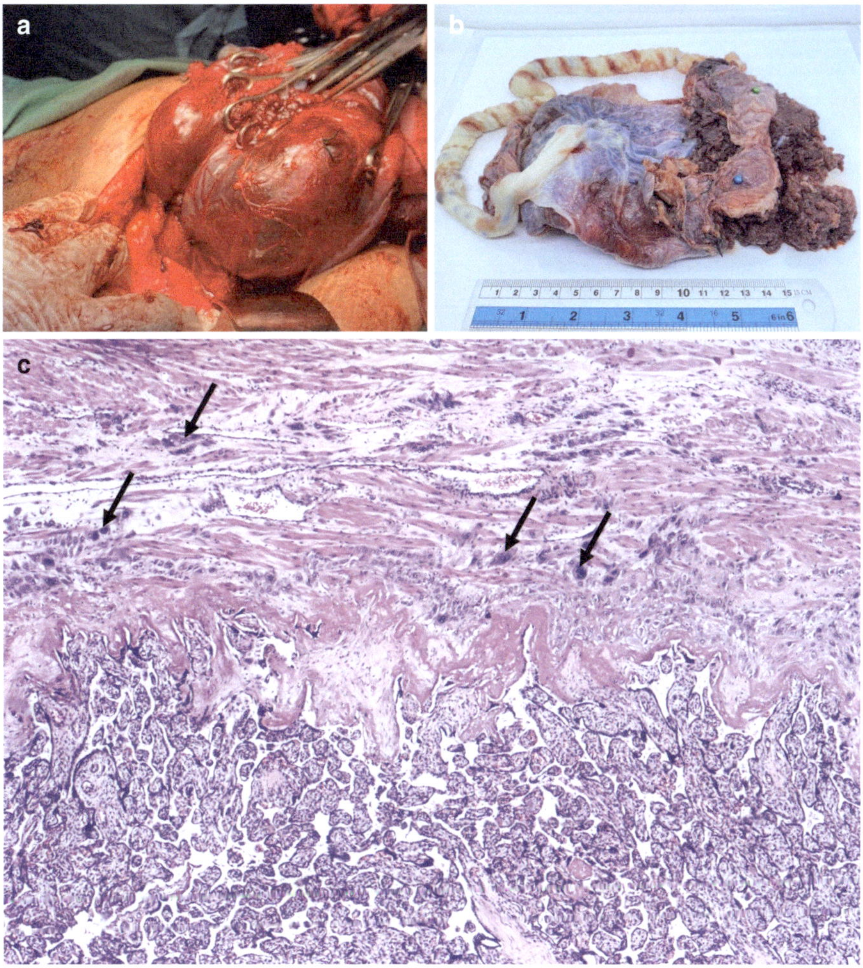

Fig. 5.2 (**a**) Bluish/purple coloring, distension (placental "bulge"); significant amounts of hypervascularity (dense tangled bed of vessels or multiple vessels running parallel craniocaudially in the uterine serosa). (**b**) Macroscopy of placenta with uterus implantation suspected placenta increta (blue and green marker). (**c**) Trophoblast extravillous within the myometrium (arrow) (Placenta increta; PAS grade 2), H&E-stained section at ×100 magnification

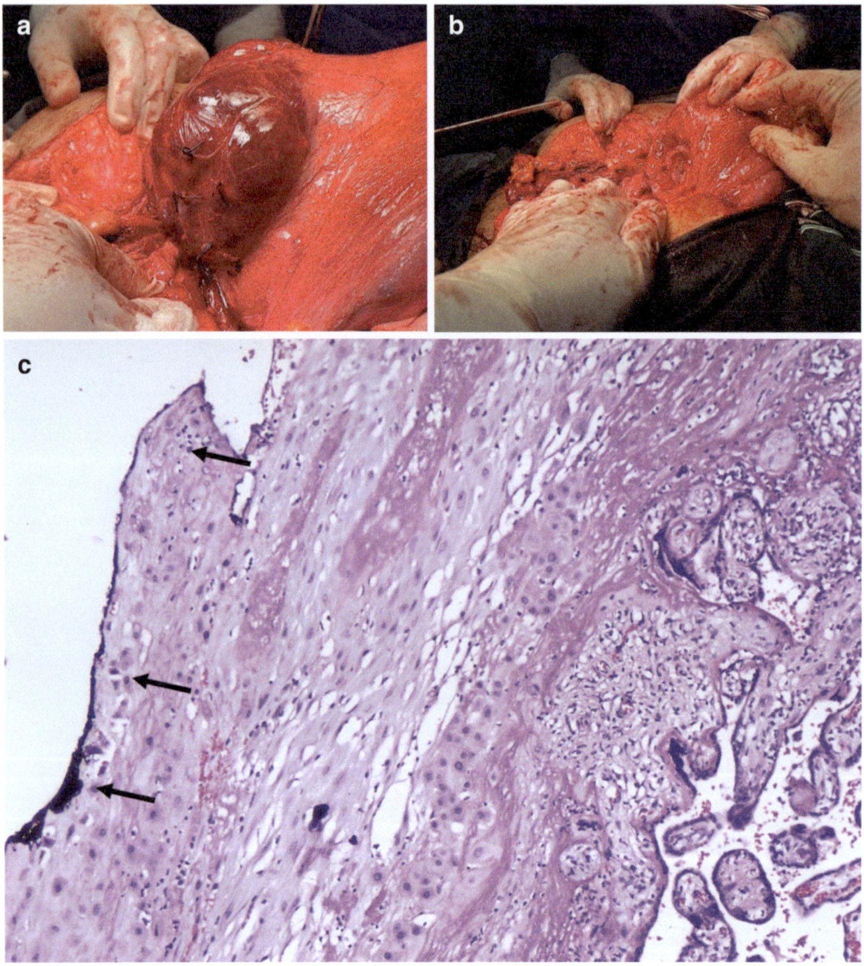

Fig. 5.3 (**a**) Serosal surface (as above) and placental tissue seen to be invading through the surface of the uterus after in the level of the above trigonal bladder after newly formed vascularies are ligated. (**b**) Local placental-myometrial resection during surgery to have sample tissue for histopathology analysis. (**c**) Trophoblast extravillous (arrow) reaching the uterine serosa (placenta percreta; PAS grade 3A) with H&E-stained section

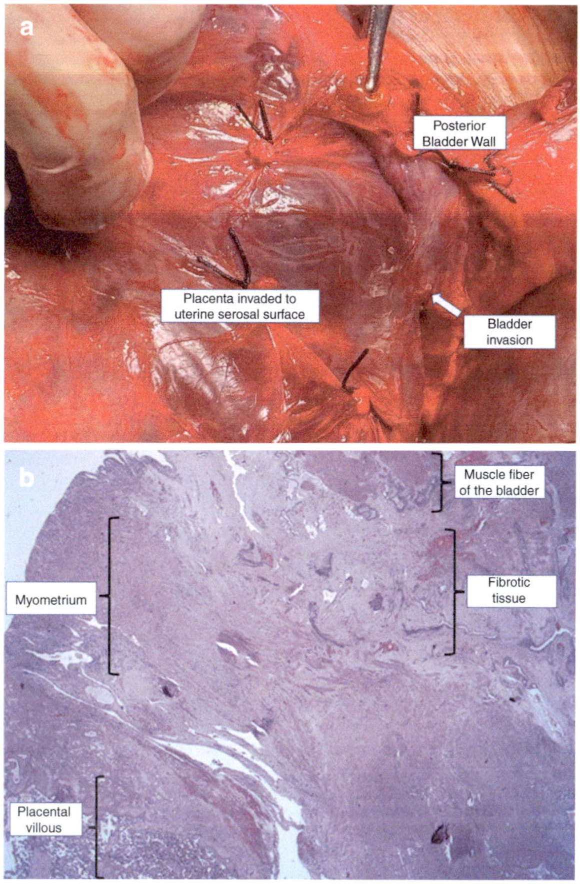

Fig. 5.4 (**a**) Clear surgical plane cannot be identified between the bladder and uterus. (**b**) Placental villi breach the uterine serosa and invade the bladder wall tissue (placenta percreta; PAS grade 3B). H&E-stained section at ×4 magnification

In Fig. 5.5, these two cases have the same grading as FIGO grade 3C but have different levels of surgical difficulties. In diffuse placental invasion, the sampling technique for histopathological examination has its challenges.

One placental invasion can have different grading of invasion and many cases of placenta accreta spectrum have both adherent and invasive areas. The separation between placental tissue from the uterine tissue in fresh specimens allowed us to differentiate between abnormally adherent and invasive areas, to evaluate the area of villous tissue invasion, and to accurately obtain a sample for histology to confirm the diagnosis of villous myometrial invasion in all cases [11, 12].

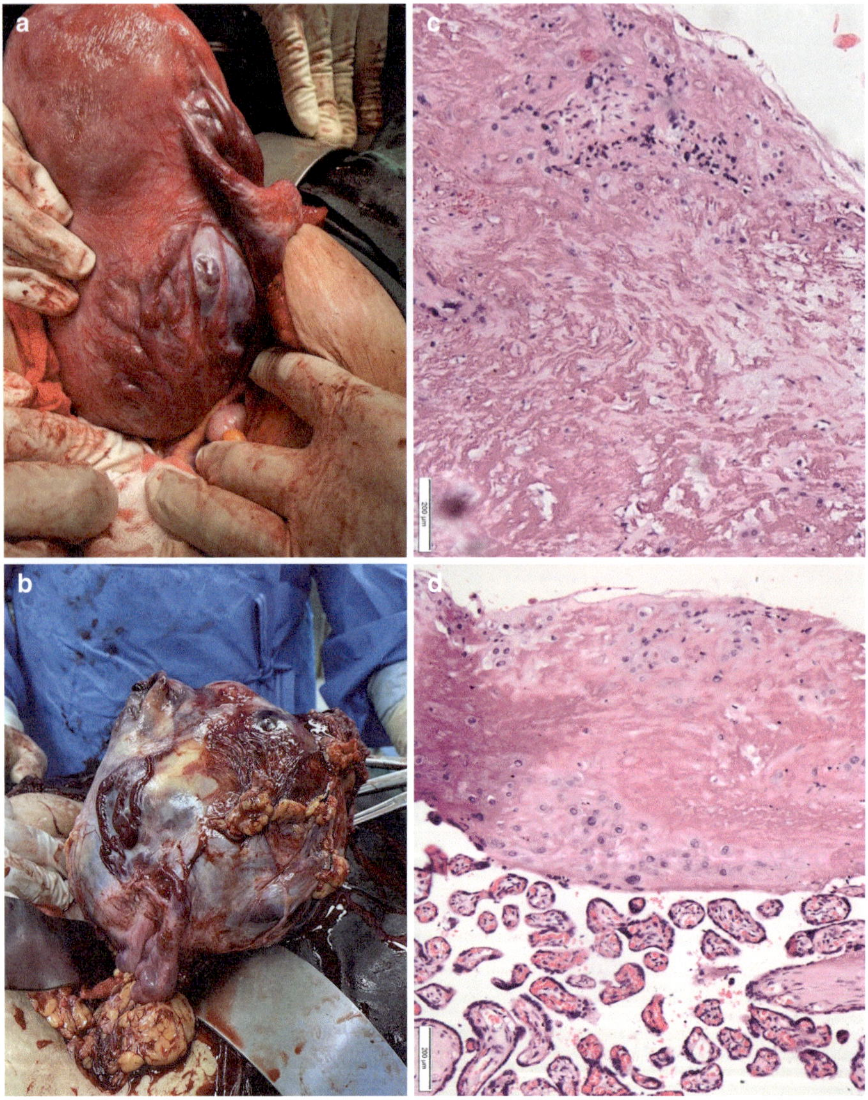

Fig. 5.5 (**a**) Placental villi are seen to be invading into the lower right parametrium with significant amounts of hypervascularity of the uterine serosa (placenta percreta; FIGO grade 3C). (**b**) Trophoblast extravillous reaching the uterine serosa with H&E-stained section. (**c**) Placental villi are seen to be invading all surfaces of right parametrium (placenta percreta; FIGO grade 3C). (**d**) Trophoblast extravillous reaching the uterine serosa with H&E-stained section

Vascular Classification

Although clinical criteria of PAS have been established by FIGO, in these criteria the difficulties at the time of PAS surgery are very difficult to describe. In clinical surgery, the level of difficulty of the surgery is strongly influenced by the location of the invasion of the placenta because it greatly affects the blood loss during surgery due to the vascular anastomoses that affect it. One of the criteria, FIGO classification of 3C with the clinical situation placenta invading through uterine serous to the parametrial-pelvic cavity, can cover upper parametrium with broad ligament and lower parametrium invasion, but these two have different prognosis due to complexity of vascular anastomosis [13].

Palacios-Jaraquemada et al. divided the uterine anastomose into S1 and S2 uterine sectors. In placental invasion above the trigonal bladder, the main vessels providing blood supply are from the uterine artery, superior vesical artery, and superior vaginal artery (Fig. 5.6a), whereas in placental invasion below the trigonal bladder, the vascular anastomoses are more complex (Fig. 5.6b) and risk of causing adverse outcomes at the time of surgery [14].

Imbalance of proangiogenic-antiangiogenic factor in PAS is the main factor that causes anastomotic vasodilation of the vascular net in the pelvic cavity area, and it depends on the degree (focal or diffuse) of placental invasion. Focal invasion shows the placenta is invading the uterine wall less than 50% of the uterine surface where diffuse invasion is more than 50% [9]. In some cases with diffuse lower PAS invasion, the vascularities are complex and the anastomosis is from extrauterine anastomosis like the branch of the rectal artery, periureteral artery, etc. [14, 15].

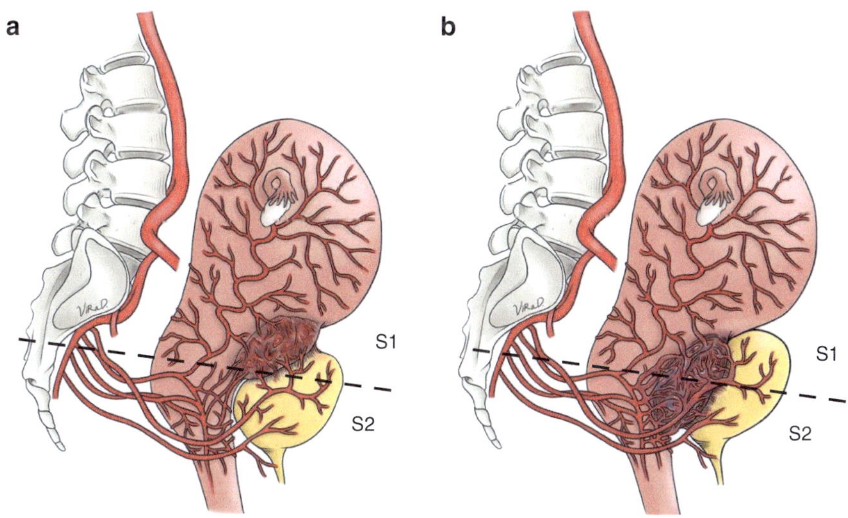

Fig. 5.6 (**a**) S1 uterine sector where the placental invasion above the trigonal bladder with major vascularities is from upper vesical-upper vaginal-uterine artery. (**b**) S2 uterine sector where the placental invasion is below the trigonal bladder which has more complex vascular anastomosis

Knowing this uterine vascular sector classification is very helpful in surgical strategies, especially the use of vascular control methods such as abdominal aortic balloon or aortic clamp [16], so this uterine sector needs to be described in detail as the surgical report for important information.

Placental-Type Invasion

The complexity of uterine vascular sector classification correlates with the location and degree of placental invasion. The other clinical classification is postponed by Palacios-Jaraquemada [17] which correlates between the complexity and the prognosis during surgery.

Type 1

This type of placental invasion is the majority of PAS which is located above the trigonal bladder and has a good prognosis for uterine resective-reconstructive surgery (Fig. 5.3a, b) [9, 17].

Type 2

The placental invasion is located in the parametrium uterine which divides the upper parametrium and lower parametrium. These two sectors have a different prognosis; lower parametrium has more complex vascularity and a high risk for maternal morbidity and mortality (Fig. 5.7) [13].

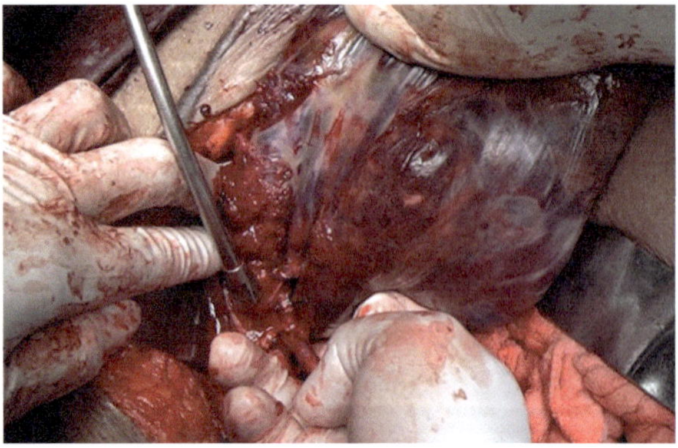

Fig. 5.7 Right lower parametrial invasion with ureter invasion

Type 3

The placenta is invaded in the lower bladder and has more complex anastomosis and lower success for uterine resective-reconstructive surgery compared with type 1 placental invasion. The importance of this type is the cervical tissue; the healthy cervix will give a higher possibility to "conserve" the uterus.

Type 4

This invasion is located in the lower bladder with massive fibrotic tissue followed by complex vascular anastomosis, and cervical invasion leads to impossible uterine resective-reconstructive surgery (lower bladder—cervical invasion).

Type 5

The placenta is invaded in the lower posterior uterus and has different vascular sources; thus, this type is more complex for vascular control. Vascular anastomosis is arrived from the branch of the superior rectal artery-inferior mesenteric artery (Fig. 5.8).

The difference between this clinical classification and the FIGO classification is that the classification relates to the prognosis and strategy at surgery, whereas the FIGO classification bridges the gap between surgical appearance and histopathology.

Both these classifications are very useful and have important meaning both during surgery and postsurgical diagnosis, so it is possible to do a combination of both classifications (Fig. 5.9).

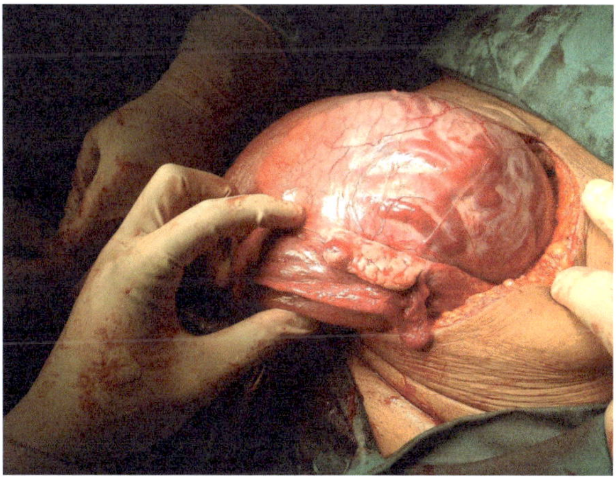

Fig. 5.8 Lower posterior invasion with a newly formed vessel from the branch of the superior rectal artery

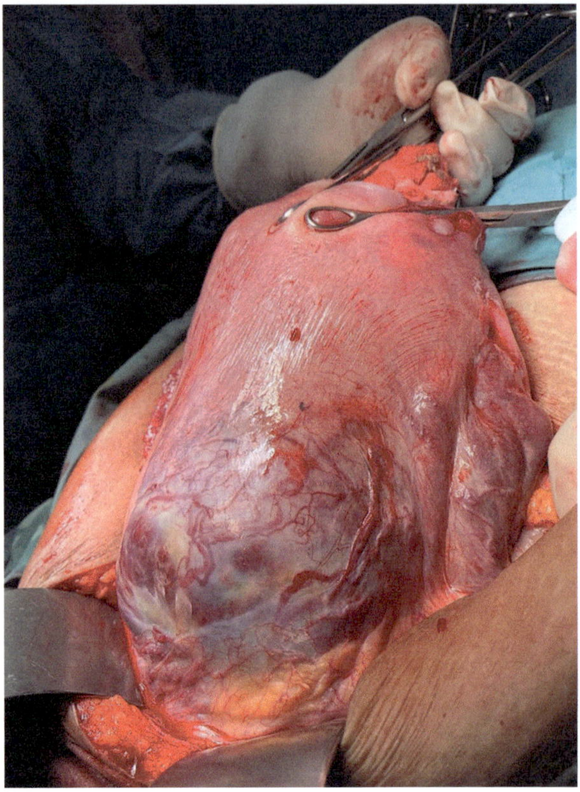

Fig. 5.9 Placenta accreta spectrum FIGO grade 3A with type 1 placental invasion—S1 uterine sector

Placental Mapping for Prenatal Diagnosis of Placenta Accreta Spectrum Grading

The concept of vascularity and placental grading is in line with the PAS pathogenesis. The placenta accreta spectrum occurs as the result of an imbalance pro-growth-inhibin factor that can lead to excessive placental invasion and vascularity growth [18].

The severity of the placenta accreta spectrum correlates with excessive angiogenesis seen on ultrasound in the form of abnormal lacunae and hypervascularity on Doppler ultrasound. The appearance of large and numerous irregular abnormal lacunae represents extensive focal or diffuse placental invasion [10, 19] (Table 5.2).

There is no single sign for ultrasound examination that is most superior because there are two things that are considered in the pre-surgical diagnosis of PAS: the depth of invasion and hypervascularity [27, 28]. The important sign which shows deep placental invasion like abnormal placental lacunae, three-dimensional power

Table 5.2 Ultrasound sign for placenta accreta spectrum [20–26]

	Ultrasound marker	Definition
Grayscale ultrasound	Loss of clear zone	Loss, or irregularity, of hypoechoic plane in myometrium underneath the placental bed ("clear zone")
	Placental bulge	Deviation of uterine serosa away from the expected plane, caused by abnormal bulge of placental tissue into neighboring organ, typically bladder; uterine serosa appears intact but outline shape is distorted
	Focal exophytic mass	Placental tissue seen breaking through uterine serosa and extending beyond it; most often seen inside filled urinary bladder
	Myometrial thinning	Thinning of myometrium overlying placenta to <1 mm or undetectable
	Bladder wall interruption	Loss or interruption in the echogenic bladder border
	Abnormal lacunae	Irregular vascular spaces within the placental parenchyma showing turbulent flow on grayscale or color doppler ultrasound
Color/power doppler ultrasound	Uterovesical hypervascularity	The presence of vessels visualized by color doppler crossing the myometrium and extending from the placenta to the posterior bladder wall or to other organs often running perpendicular to myometrium
	Subplacental hypervascularity	Striking amount of color doppler signal seen in placental bed; this sign probably indicates numerous, closely packed, tortuous vessels in that region (demonstrating multidirectional flow and aliasing artifact)
	Bridging vessel	Vessels appearing to extend from placenta, across myometrium, and beyond serosa into bladder or other organs; often running perpendicular to myometrium
	Placental lacunae feeding vessel	Vessels with high-velocity blood flow leading from myometrium into placental lacunae, causing turbulence upon entry
	Parametrial invasion	Placental bulge in the parametrial region with sign of hypervascularity
3D rendering-3D doppler ultrasound	Three-dimensional rendering ultrasound	Disconnection of two parallel lines in uteroplacental-bladder interface
	Three-dimensional power doppler ultrasound	Intraplacental vascularization and vascularization of uterine serosa-bladder interface
Other sign	"Rail sign"	The parallel subplacental/uterovesical hypervascularity, and neovascularization of the bladder mucosa, together with interconnected bridging vessels
	Transvaginal ultrasound: Intracervical lacunae	Tortuous anechoic space within the cervix which appeared hypervascular at color doppler

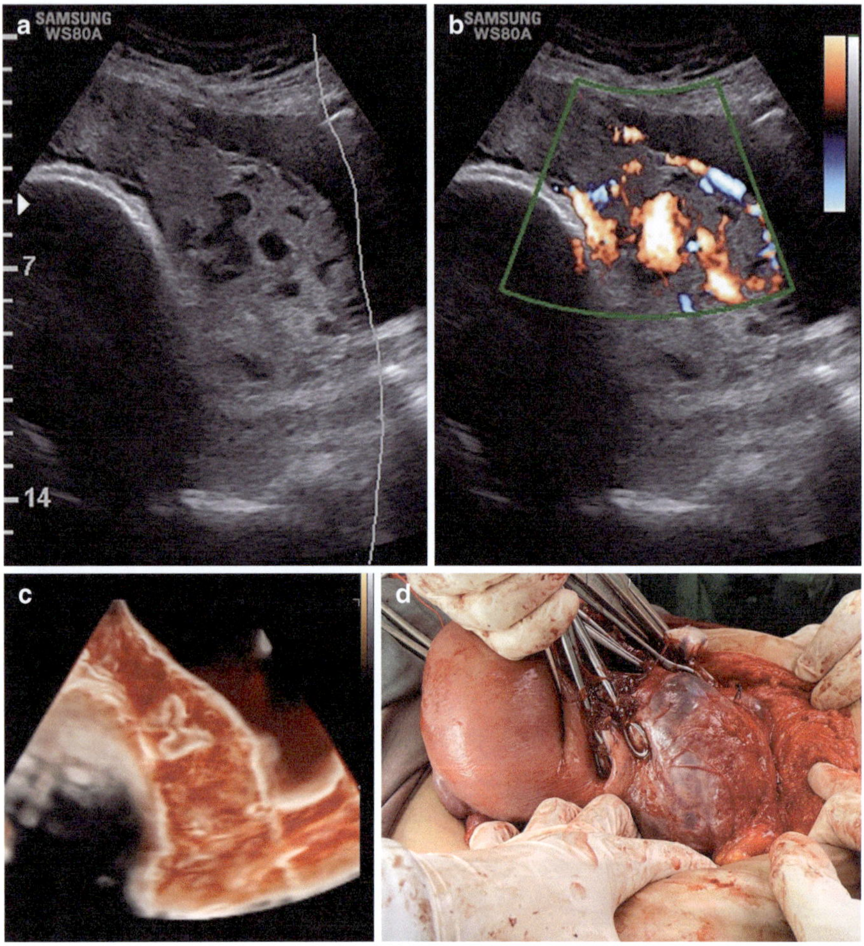

Fig. 5.10 (**a**) Grayscale ultrasound shows loss of clear zone, abnormal lacunae, placental bulge, and bladder wall interruption. (**b**) Color Doppler shows uterovesical hypervascularity, bridging vessel, and rail sign. (**c**) 3D rendering ultrasound shows loss of two parallel lines in uteroplacental-bladder interface with the placental tissue attached in the bladder wall which gives impression for highly suspicious lower bladder invasion. (**d**) Bladder invasion of PAS FIGO grade 3B with type 4 placental invasion—S2 uterine sector

Doppler ultrasound, and rail sign can help to know the deepest placental invasion (Fig. 5.10) [22, 23, 25].

The concept of S1/S2 uterine sector is very useful in pre-surgical diagnostic examination to know the possibility for uterine resective-reconstructive surgery. Lower bladder invasion can be evaluated using three-dimensional ultrasound or transvaginal ultrasound to analyze the cervical hypervascularity and cervical lacunae (Fig. 5.11). This concept is very important because high-grade PAS usually

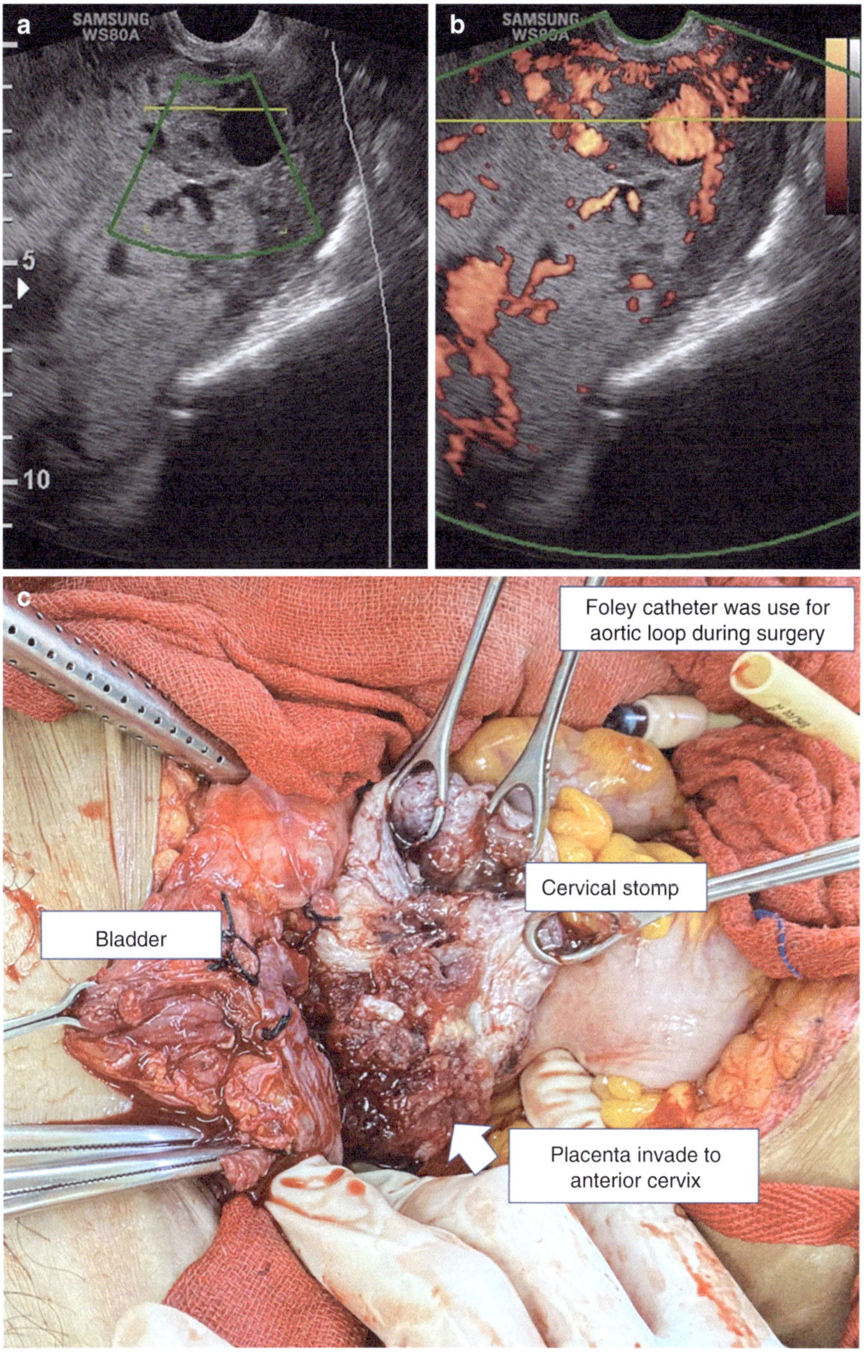

Fig. 5.11 (**a**) Transvaginal ultrasound shows the placenta invading the anterior cervix with abnormal lacunae. (**b**) Cervical hypervascularity and intracervical lacunae show S2 uterine sector of uteroplacental vascularity. (**c**) Cervical invasion (white arrow) during modified subtotal hysterectomy with abdominal aortic loop using Foley catheter

has correlation with lower invasion due to complex vascular anastomosis where aortic control may preferable to control the bleeding during surgery [16, 24, 26, 29].

Conclusion

The concept of classification of placenta accreta spectrum (PAS) is bridging the pre-, intra-, and postsurgical diagnosis. Combining classification between FIGO classification, placental invasion type, and S1/S2 uterine sector may useful for surgical strategies and sampling of placental tissue for histopathology and should be considered during placental mapping of ultrasound examination especially for advanced grading of PAS.

References

1. Jauniaux E, Bhide A, Kennedy A, Woodward P, Hubinont C, Collins S, et al. FIGO consensus guidelines on placenta accreta spectrum disorders: prenatal diagnosis and screening. Int J Gynecol Obstet. 2018;140(3):274–80.
2. Silver RM. Abnormal placentation: placenta previa, vasa previa, and placenta accreta. Obstet Gynecol. 2015;126:3.
3. Morlando M, Collins S. Placenta accreta spectrum disorders: challenges, risks, and management strategies. Int J Women's Health. 2020;12:1033–45.
4. Bhide A, Sebire N, Abuhamad A, Acharya G, Silver R. Morbidly adherent placenta: the need for standardization. Ultrasound Obstet Gynecol. 2017;49:559–63.
5. Irving FC, Hertig AT. A study of placenta accreta. Surg Gynecol Obstet. 1937;64:178–200.
6. Fox H. Placenta Accreta, 1945–1969. Obstet Gynecol Surv. 1972;27:7.
7. Jauniaux E, Grønbeck L, Bunce C, Langhoff-Roos J, Collins SL. Epidemiology of placenta previa accreta: a systematic review and meta-analysis. BMJ Open. 2019;9(11):e031193.
8. Jauniaux E, Collins S, Burton GJ. Placenta accreta spectrum: pathophysiology and evidence-based anatomy for prenatal ultrasound imaging. Am J Obstet Gynecol. 2018;218(1):75–87.
9. Palacios Jaraquemada JM, Pesaresi M, Nassif JC, Hermosid S. Anterior placenta percreta: surgical approach, hemostasis and uterine repair. Acta Obstet Gynecol Scand. 2004;83(8):738–44.
10. Dannheim K, Shainker SA, Hecht JL. Hysterectomy for placenta accreta; methods for gross and microscopic pathology examination. Arch Gynecol Obstet. 2016;293(5):951–8.
11. Jauniaux E, Hussein AM, Fox KA, Collins SL. New evidence-based diagnostic and management strategies for placenta accreta spectrum disorders. Best Pract Res Clin Obstet Gynaecol. 2019;61:75–88.
12. Jauniaux E, Hussein AM, Zosmer N, Elbarmelgy RM, Elbarmelgy RA, Shaikh H, et al. A new methodologic approach for clinico-pathologic correlations in invasive placenta previa accreta. Am J Obstet Gynecol. 2020;222(4):379.e1–379.e11.
13. Palacios-Jaraquemada JM, D'Antonio F, Buca D, Fiorillo A, Larraza P. Systematic review on near miss cases of placenta accreta spectrum disorders: correlation with invasion topography, prenatal imaging, and surgical outcome. J Matern Neonatal Med. 2020;33(19):3377–84.
14. Palacios Jaraquemada JM, Garcia Monaco R, Barbosa NE, Ferle L, Iriarte H, Conesa HA. Lower uterine blood supply: extrauterine anastomotic system and its application in surgical devascularization techniques. Acta Obstet Gynecol Scand. 2007;86(2):228–34.

15. Palacios-Jaraquemada JM, D'Antonio F, Buca D, Fiorillo A, Larraza P. Systematic review on near miss cases of placenta accreta spectrum disorders: correlation with invasion topography, prenatal imaging, and surgical outcome. J Matern Fetal Neonatal Med. 2019:1–8.
16. Nieto-Calvache AJ, Palacios-Jaraquemada JM, Aryananda RA. Factors to consider when seeking better results in placenta accreta spectrum. Acta Obstet Gynecol Scand. 2021;100(10):1932–3.
17. Palacios-Jaraquemada JM, Fiorillo A, Hamer J, Martinez M, Bruno C. Placenta accreta spectrum: a hysterectomy can be prevented in almost 80% of cases using a resective-reconstructive technique. J Matern Fetal Neonatal Med. 2020:1–8.
18. Bartels HC, Postle JD, Downey P, Brennan DJ. Placenta accreta spectrum: a review of pathology, molecular biology, and biomarkers. Rebelo I, editor. Dis Markers. 2018;2018:1507674.
19. Jauniaux E, Zosmer N, Subramanian D, Shaikh H, Burton GJ. Ultrasound-histopathologic features of the utero-placental interface in placenta accreta spectrum. Placenta. 2020;97:58–64.
20. Collins SL, Ashcroft A, Braun T, Calda P, Langhoff-Roos J, Morel O, et al. Proposal for standardized ultrasound descriptors of abnormally invasive placenta (AIP). Ultrasound Obstet Gynecol. 2016;47:271–5.
21. Alfirevic Z, Tang A-W, Collins SL, Robson SC, Palacios-Jaraquemada J. Pro forma for ultrasound reporting in suspected abnormally invasive placenta (AIP): an international consensus. Ultrasound Obstet Gynecol. 2016;47:276–8.
22. Shih JC, Palacios Jaraquemada JMP, Su YN, Shyu MK, Lin CH, Lin SY, et al. Role of three-dimensional power Doppler in the antenatal diagnosis of placenta accreta: comparison with gray-scale and color Doppler techniques. Ultrasound Obstet Gynecol. 2009;33(2):193–203.
23. Cali G, Foti F, Minneci G. 3D power Doppler in the evaluation of abnormally invasive placenta. J Perinat Med. 2017;45(6):701–9.
24. di Pasquo E, Ghi T, Calì G, D'Antonio F, Fratelli N, Forlani F, et al. Intracervical lakes as sonographic marker of placenta accreta spectrum disorder in patients with placenta previa or low-lying placenta. Ultrasound Obstet Gynecol. 2020;55(4):460–6.
25. Shih J-C, Kang J, Tsai S-J, Lee J-K, Liu K-L, Huang K-Y. The "rail sign" : an ultrasound finding in placenta accreta spectrum indicating deep villous invasion and adverse outcomes. Am J Obstet Gynecol. 2021;
26. Aryananda RA, Akbar A, Wardhana MP, Gumilar KE, Wicaksono B, Ernawati E, et al. New three-dimensional/four-dimensional volume rendering imaging software for detecting the abnormally invasive placenta. J Clin Ultrasound. 2019;47:1.
27. Cali G, Forlani F, Timor Trisch I, Palacios-Jaraquemada J, Foti F, Minneci G, et al. Diagnostic accuracy of ultrasound in detecting the depth of invasion in women at risk of abnormally invasive placenta: a prospective longitudinal study. Acta Obstet Gynecol Scand. 2018;97(10):1219–27.
28. Pagani G, Cali G, Acharya G, Trisch I-T, Palacios-Jaraquemada J, Familiari A, et al. Diagnostic accuracy of ultrasound in detecting the severity of abnormally invasive placentation: a systematic review and meta-analysis. Acta Obstet Gynecol Scand. 2018;97(1):25–37.
29. Cali G, Forlani F, Lees C, Timor-Tritsch I, Palacios-Jaraquemada J, Dall'Asta A, et al. Prenatal ultrasound staging system for placenta accreta spectrum disorders. Ultrasound Obstet Gynecol. 2019;53(6):752–60.

Chapter 6
Diagnosis of Placenta Accreta Spectrum: Clinical and Radiological Diagnosis of Placenta Accreta Spectrum and the Ability of Sonographic and MRI Findings to Predict Definitive Diagnosis

Bahram Salmanian, Scott A. Shainker, Alireza A. Shamshirsaz, and Ahmed A. Nassr

The Importance of Antenatal Diagnosis of Placenta Accreta Spectrum

Placenta accreta spectrum (PAS) is a morbid complication of pregnancy that results from abnormal placentation. In normal pregnancies, the placenta implants in the decidua functionalis and does not adhere to deeper tissue. It is suggested that the partial or complete lack of decidua basalis results in deeper penetration of the placenta into myometrium. Placental growth may be limited to the endometrium (accreta), to myometrium (increta), or through the uterine serosa (percreta) with possible involvement of the adjacent organs. As the cesarean delivery rate increases, there has been a significant increase in the incidence of PAS. In the United States, the incidence increased from 1 in 30,000 pregnancies in 1960s to 1 in 2500 pregnancies in the 1990s [1] and further increased to 1 in 533 pregnancies in the early 2000s [2]; however, the true incidence of PAS is unknown as the reported rates vary when outside of research protocols [3].

B. Salmanian · A. A. Shamshirsaz · A. A. Nassr (✉)
Department of Obstetrics and Gynecology, Baylor College of Medicine and Texas Children's Hospital, Houston, TX, USA
e-mail: Ahmed.Nassr@bcm.edu

S. A. Shainker
New England Center for Placental Disorders, Beth Israel Deaconess Medical Center, Boston, MA, USA

Department of Obstetrics, Gynecology, and Reproductive Biology, Harvard Medical School, Boston, MA, USA

S. A. Shazly, A. A. Nassr (eds.), *Placenta Accreta Spectrum*,
https://doi.org/10.1007/978-3-031-10347-6_6

Clinically, the major risk factors for PAS are history of prior cesarean delivery and presence of placenta previa in the current pregnancy. The risk significantly increases with history of multiple cesarean deliveries [4–6]. Other risk factors include prior uterine surgery other than cesarean [7–9], assisted reproduction [10, 11], advanced maternal age [12], and multiple gestation [13, 14].

The predominant morbidity associated with PAS is obstetric hemorrhage, often requiring multiple units of blood products and possible complications with massive transfusion [15–18]. Due to the complexity of surgery at the time of delivery, often accompanied with hysterectomy, surgical complications are common with PAS including bladder and ureteral injury, or other adjacent organs in the pelvis.

Maternal outcomes are improved when there is antenatal diagnosis prior to delivery, allowing for advanced planning and multidisciplinary management of PAS to achieve favorable outcomes [19, 20]. This reflects the importance of accurate diagnostic tools particularly in the high-risk population to avoid poor outcomes. PAS evaluation should be considered in any pregnancy with placenta previa and history of cesarean delivery. Antepartum diagnosis helps with planning the delivery under optimized conditions in experienced centers.

Antenatal Diagnosis: Role of Different Imaging Modalities

Definitive diagnosis is by histopathologic evaluation of the placenta and the uterus. However, imaging techniques are available that can predict PAS with good accuracy. The sensitivity of ultrasound in the diagnosis of PAS is reported to be 90.7% (95% CI, 87.2–93.6) with specificity of 96.9% (95% CI, 96.3–97.5%) [21]. However, the experience of the operator and clinician reading the ultrasound images may affect the accuracy. In addition, recent study suggests intraoperative clinical diagnosis correlate well with pathologic diagnosis [22].

In 1982, the first documented antenatal diagnosis of PAS was reported [23]. Since then several markers are introduced to improve the accuracy of PAS diagnosis on imaging. Advances in technology also have helped for better visualization and description of various markers and findings. Ultrasound is the modality of choice for the evaluation of the placenta. It is safe during pregnancy, it provides easy availability with real-time assessment, and it is the cheapest diagnostic imaging available compared to other tools such as MRI. There have been recent efforts to establish a standardized protocol for ultrasound evaluation of PAS in relation to clinical and pathological findings. There are several sonographic markers associated with PAS, and some can be seen as early as the first trimester pregnancy. For all pregnancies, standard of care is to evaluate placental location and implantation universally during the midtrimester anatomy scan. Magnetic resonance imaging (MRI) can also help when placenta cannot clearly be visualized on ultrasound or the findings are not conclusive. There are scoring systems introduced for antenatal assessment of PAS involving both clinical risk factors and US markers [24–26]. The presence of placenta previa in patients with history of prior cesarean delivery has the most influence in these scoring systems suggested.

First Trimester Imaging

Early in pregnancy, a gestational sac implanted in the lower uterine segment in close proximity to the previous uterine scar increases the risk of PAS [27, 28]. It has been reported that 28% of patients with PAS have low implantation of the gestational sac on the first trimester ultrasound [28]. Cesarean section scar pregnancy is a marker for PAS, and all the sonographic PAS markers described on a second or third trimester ultrasound can also be seen on a first trimester scan [29], including as anechoic placental areas and an irregular uteroplacental interface (Fig. 6.1) [30]. Particularly concerning for early PAS is when the residual myometrial thickness is less than 5 mm at the implantation site within the previous cesarean scar; this finding increases the risk for need for hysterectomy if the pregnancy continues [28]. In case of cesarean scar pregnancy, there are studies reporting a new sonographic sign (the crossover sign or COS) that can predict the severity of subsequent PAS and possibility of a successful pregnancy [31]. The COS is a measure of the relationship between the gestational sac, anterior uterine wall, and cesarean scar.

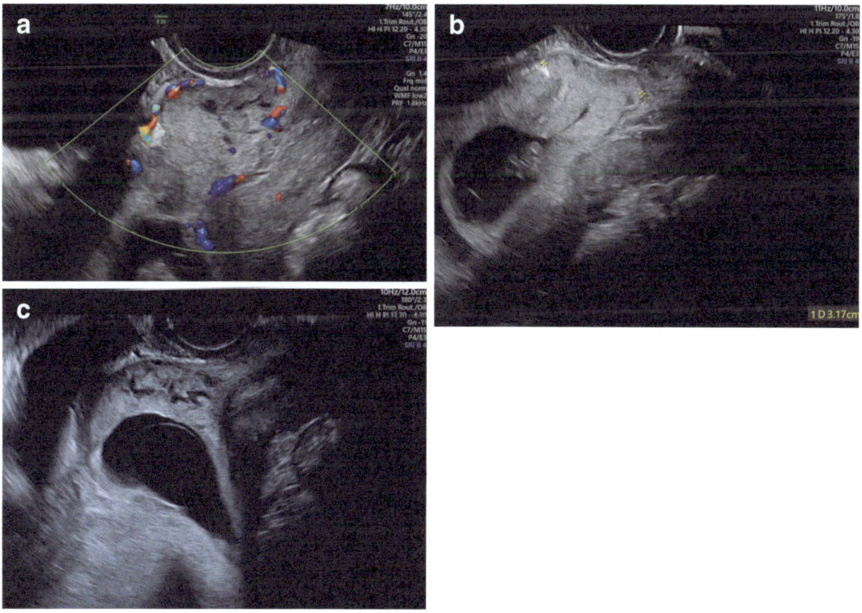

Fig. 6.1 Ultrasound images of a first trimester pregnancy with cesarean scar implantation; (**a**, **b**) sagittal image of the lower uterine segment with extension of the decidua into the myometrium at 8 weeks; (**c**) sagittal image of the same pregnancy at 9 weeks with formation of lacunae

Second or Third Trimester Ultrasound Evaluation

There are multiple ultrasound markers associated with PAS in the second or third trimester [26, 32]. Most of these markers are present at the time of midtrimester anatomy scan. Transvaginal sonography with a partially full urinary bladder is in particular recommended for evaluation of the lower uterine segment and vesicouterine interface [33]. Color Doppler is the other imaging tool that can be helpful and should be used to visualize PAS-associated vascular abnormalities.

These markers include (Fig. 6.2) the following:

1. Placenta lacunae: hypoechoic spaces with irregular margins within the placental tissue visible on gray scale; color Doppler often reveals a swirling of venous flow. The following criteria are associated with high-risk PAS:

   - Multiple lesions (>3).
   - Large size.
   - Irregular borders.
   - High velocity and/or turbulent flow within.

     In patients who are higher risk for PAS with history of prior cesarean delivery and placenta previa, absence of lacunae has negative predictive values (NPV) ranging from 88% to 100% [34, 35].

2. Irregular uteroplacental interface includes the loss of the retroplacental hypoechoic zone between the placenta and myometrium as well as thinning of the retroplacental myometrium (<1 mm):

   - This marker should be evaluated particularly along the posterior bladder wall; a partial or complete interruption of the uterovesical interface can often be seen.
   - It is important to ensure the correct angle of insonation and avoid undue pressure on the abdomen or with the transvaginal ultrasound probe as this has been shown to obscure imaging accuracy [36].

3. Uterine wall bulging as a result of placental tissue distorting uterine contour.
4. Placental extrusion beyond the uterine wall:

   - This marker can represent uterine wall dehiscence as well.

5. Bridging vessels:

   - Placental vasculature crossing from the placenta into the myometrium (and sometimes beyond).
   - Neovascularization at the placental implantation/invasion site is often represented as vessels crossing the uterine serosa into uterovesical space or other adjacent anatomic planes [37].
   - Attention is required to distinguish lower uterine segment hypervascularity often associated with placenta previa from bridging vessels.

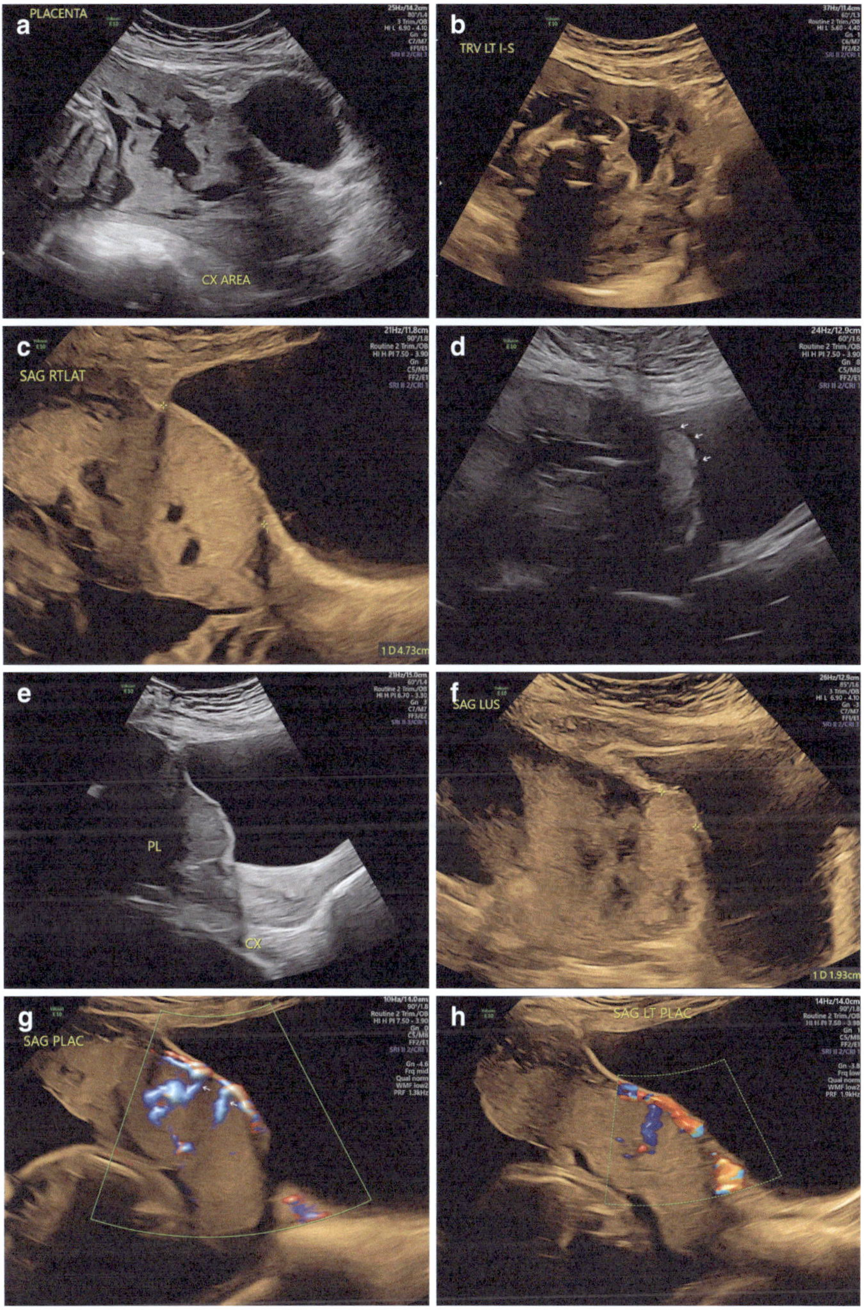

Fig. 6.2 Ultrasound markers of placenta accreta spectrum on images of lower uterine segment; (**a**) sagittal view with placenta lacunae present; (**b**) transverse view with placenta lacunae present; (**c**) loss of the retroplacental hypoechoic zone between the placenta and myometrium; (**d**, **e**). sagittal view with irregular uteroplacental interface and bulging of the placenta toward the bladder with loss of the retroplacental hypoechoic zone between the placenta and myometrium; (**f**) sagittal view of placental extrusion beyond the uterine wall into the bladder; (**g**, **h**) sagittal view of hypervascularity of the placenta myometrium interface with bridging vessels

If PAS is suspected, the extent of placental involvement, focal or global, and the depth of placental invasion, confined to the uterus or extending to the adjacent organs such as the bladder or parametrium, should also be evaluated.

There are other techniques that can help to improve diagnosis but are not well described yet. Measurement of the peak systolic velocity of placental vasculature has been shown to have a direct correlation with PAS; however, it lacks sensitivity with a low negative predictive value [38]. Three-dimensional (3D) US in combination with power Doppler may also help to better evaluate the placental-myometrial interface looking for hypervascularity, and tortuous vascularity with chaotic branching, and also help to better evaluate for involvement of adjacent organs [39]. Detection of hypervascularity of the uterine-bladder interface by 3D ultrasound is reported to have superior diagnostic sensitivity and specificity over 2D imaging with 100% positive predictive value [40]. However, 3D imaging remains a complex technique requiring operator expertise and may not be an available option in some centers.

It should be taken into account that the presence of these markers in the low-risk population without placenta previa or history of previous cesarean delivery may be hard to interpret and often does not convey an increased risk for PAS [41].

MRI Evaluation

Additional MRI can provide similar diagnostic accuracy when compared to ultrasound. Due to the higher cost of MRI, it is recommended to consider MRI when ultrasound evaluation of the placenta is technically difficult such as in posterior placentation, morbid obesity, or multiple gestation [42]. Other limiting factors for US evaluation are operator dependency, quality of equipment used, and acoustic effects such as fetal position, prior scars, uterine contraction, myomas, and insufficient or excessive maternal urinary bladder filling. Overall, MRI provides similar detection rate compared to US for PAS diagnosis [42, 43]; however, it can provide more details regarding the depth of invasion and adjacent organ involvement [26, 44].

T2-weighted imaging is the modality for placental evaluation. The MRI markers for PAS include (Fig. 6.3):

1. Dark intraplacental bands.
2. Heterogenous signal intensity in the placenta.
3. Focal areas of uterine bulging.
4. Loss of the interface with adjacent organs.

Of the above markers, the first two are the most sensitive and the latter two are the most specific findings for PAS [45].

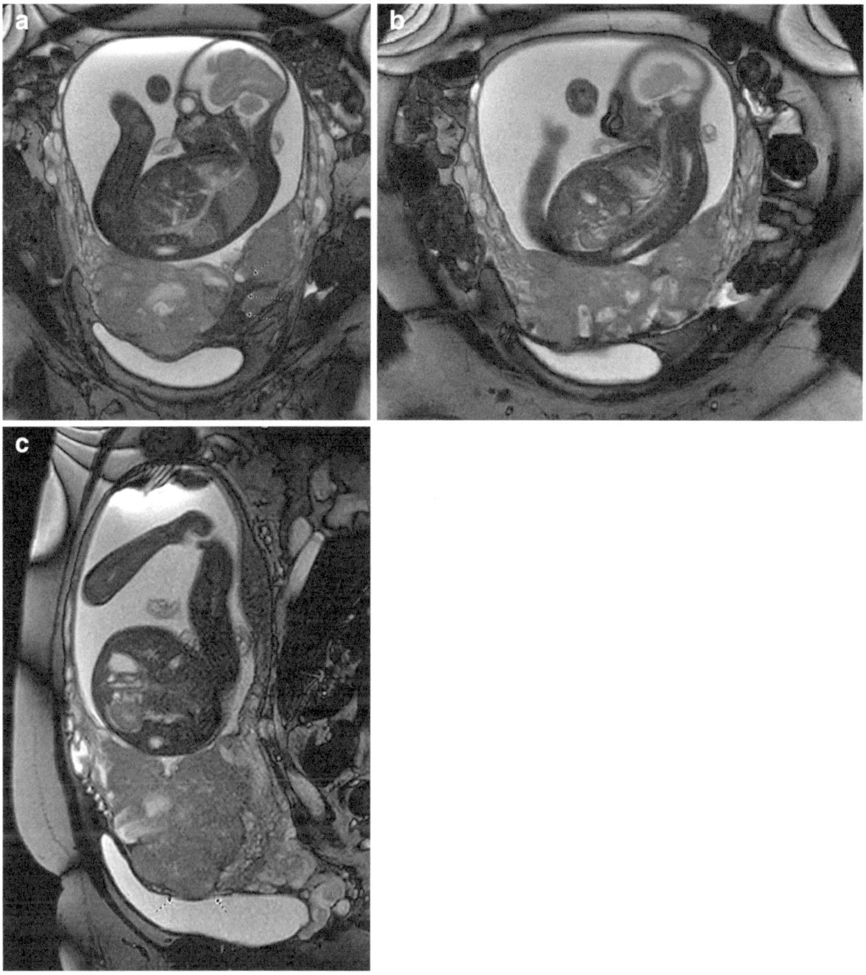

Fig. 6.3 Magnetic resonance imaging and markers for placenta accreta spectrum; (**a**, **b**) dark intraplacental bands with heterogenous signal intensity in the placenta; (**c**) focal areas of uterine bulging

Other MRI markers include thick T2-hypointense septa within the myometrium likely due to myometrial invasion, tenting of the urinary bladder, and abnormal vascular formation in the placenta as tortuous and enlarged spaces on T2-weighted sequence [45].

It is recommended that at least two of the above findings should be present to raise concern for PAS [46, 47]. MRI has sensitivity and specificity increases after 24 weeks of gestation, up to 79% and 94%, respectively [48]. Although MRI is overall safe in pregnancy, use of gadolinium-based intravenous contrast is not recommended for possible fetal side effects [49, 50].

Special Considerations

- Despite ongoing efforts to improve antenatal diagnosis of PAS, PAS is often not diagnosed until the time of delivery. Under such circumstances, when appropriate resources for managing such patients are not available, temporary closure of the abdomen and rapid transfer to a tertiary center with higher level of care can be considered as long as the patient is hemodynamically stable.
- False-positive diagnosis of PAS may introduce unnecessary perinatal morbidity. However, a recent study investigating the outcomes in such patients revealed acceptable outcomes if managed in a referral center with expertise in managing PAS. The incidence of unnecessary hysterectomy was reported to be 2% or less [51].

References

1. Miller DA, Vhollet JA, Goodwin TM. Clinical risk factors for placenta previa-placenta accreta. Am J Obstet Gynecol. 1997;177:210–4.
2. Wu S, Kocherginsky M, Hibbard JU. Abnormal placentation: twenty-year analysis. Am J Obstet Gynecol. 2005;192:1458–61.
3. Bailit JL, Grobman WA, Rice MM, Reddy UM, Wapner RJ, Varner MW, et al. Eunice Kennedy Shriver National Institute of Child Health and Human Development (NICHD) Maternal Fetal Medicine Units (MFMU) Network. Morbidly adherent placenta treatments and outcomes. Obstet Gynecol. 2015;125(3):683–9.
4. Clark SL, Koonings PP, Phelan JP. Placenta previa/accreta and prior cesarean section. Obstet Gynecol. 1985;66:89–92.
5. Silver RM, Landon MB, Rouse DJ, Leveno KJ, Spong CY, Thom EA, et al. Maternal morbidity associated with multiple repeat cesarean deliveries. Obstet Gynecol. 2006;107:1226–32.
6. Erfani H, Fox KA, Clark SL, Rac M, Rocky Hui SK, Rezaei A, Aalipour S, Shamshirsaz AA, Nassr AA, Salmanian B, Stewart KA, Kravitz ES, Eppes C, Coburn M, Espinoza J, Teruya J, Belfort MA, Shamshirsaz AA. Maternal outcomes in unexpected placenta accreta spectrum disorders: single-center experience with a multidisciplinary team. Am J Obstet Gynecol. 2019;221(4):337.e1–5.
7. Gyamfi-Bannerman C, Gilbert S, Landon MB, Spong CY, Rouse DJ, Varner MW, et al. Risk of uterine rupture and placenta accreta with prior uterine surgery outside of the lower segment. Obstet Gynecol. 2012;120:1332–7.
8. Kohn JR, Shamshirsaz AA, Popek E, Guan X, Belfort MA, Fox KA. Pregnancy after endometrial ablation: a systematic review. BJOG. 2018;125(1):43–53.
9. Carusi DA, Fox KA, Lyell DJ, Perlman NC, Aalipour S, Einerson BD, Belfort MA, Silver RM, Shamshirsaz AA. Placenta accreta spectrum without placenta previa. Obstet Gynecol. 2020;136(3):458–65.
10. Salmanian B, Fox KA, Arian SE, Erfani H, Clark SL, Aagaard KM, Detlefs SE, Aalipour S, Espinoza J, Nassr AA, Gibbons WE, Shamshirsaz AA, Belfort MA, Shamshirsaz AA. In vitro fertilization as an independent risk factor for placenta accreta spectrum. Am J Obstet Gynecol. 2020;223(4):568.e1–5.
11. Modest AM, Toth TL, Johnson KM, Shainker SA. Placenta accreta spectrum: in vitro fertilization and non-in vitro fertilization and placenta Accreta Spectrum in a Massachusetts Cohort. Am J Perinatol. 2021;38(14):1533–9.
12. Miller DA, Chollet JA, Goodwin TM. Clinical risk factors for placenta previa and placenta accreta. Am J Obstet Gynecol. 1997;177(1):210–4.

13. Shamshirsaz AA, Carusi D, Shainker SA, Einerson B, Khandelwal M, Erfani H, Shamshirsaz AA, Modest AM, Aalipour S, Fox KA, Lyell DJ, Belfort MA, Silver RM. Characteristics and outcomes of placenta accreta spectrum in twins versus singletons: a study from the pan American Society for Placenta Accreta Spectrum (PAS(2)). Am J Obstet Gynecol. 2020;222(6):624–5.
14. Miller HE, Leonard SA, Fox KA, Carusi DA, Lyell DJ. Placenta accreta spectrum among women with twin gestations. Obstet Gynecol. 2020:3. Online ahead of print
15. Fitzpatrick KE, Sellers S, Spark P, Kurinczuk JJ, Brocklehurst P, Knight M. The management and outcomes of placenta accreta, increta, and percreta in the UK: a population-based descriptive study. BJOG. 2014;121(1):62–70.
16. Wright JD, Pri-Paz S, Herzog TJ, Shah M, Bonanno C, Lewin SN, et al. Predictors of massive blood loss in women with placenta accreta. Am J Obstet Gynecol. 2011;205(38):e1–6.
17. Eller AG, Porter TF, Soisson P, Silver RM. Optimal management strategies for placenta accreta. BJOG. 2009;116:648–54.
18. Warshak CR, Ramos GA, Eskander R, Benirschke K, Saenz CC, Kelly TF, et al. Effect of predelivery diagnosis in 99 consecutive cases of placenta accreta. Obstet Gynecol. 2010;115:65–9.
19. Shamshiraz AA, Fox KA, Salmanian B, Diaz-Arrastia CR, Lee W, Baker BW, et al. Maternal morbidity in patients with morbidly adherent placenta treated with and without a standardized multidisciplinary approach. Am J Obstet Gynecol. 2015;212(218):e1–9.
20. Shamshirsaz AA, Fox KA, Erfani H, et al. Multidisciplinary team learning in the management of the morbidly adherent placenta: outcome improvements over time. Am J Obstet Gynecol. 2017;216(612):e1–5.
21. D'Antonio F, Iacovella C, Bhide A. Prenatal identification of invasive placentation using ultrasound: systematic review and meta-analysis. Ultrasound Obstet Gynecol. 2013;42(5):509–17.
22. Salmanian B, Shainker SA, Hecht JL, Modest AM, Castro EC, Seaman RD, Meshinchiasl N, Hessami K, Brown A, Tounsi S, Shamshirsaz AA, Fox KA, Clark SL, Belfort MA, Shamshirsaz AA. The Society for Pediatric Pathology Task Force grading system for placenta accreta spectrum and its correlation with clinical outcomes. Am J Obstet Gynecol. 2022; S0002-9378(22)00100-4
23. Tabsh KM, Brinkman CR 3rd, King W. Ultrasound diagnosis of placenta increta. J Clin Ultrasound. 1982;10(6):288–90.
24. Jauniaux E, Kingdom JC, Silver RM. A comparison of recent guidelines in the diagnosis and management of placenta accreta spectrum disorders. Best Pract Res Clin Obstet Gynaecol. 2020;
25. Jauniaux E, Bhide A. Prenatal ultrasound diagnosis and outcome of placenta previa accreta after cesarean delivery: a systematic review and meta-analysis. Am J Obstet Gynecol. 2017;217(1):27–36.
26. Pagani G, Cali G, Acharya G, et al. Diagnostic accuracy of ultrasound in detecting the severity of abnormally invasive placentation: a systematic review and meta-analysis. Acta Obstet Gynecol Scand. 2018;97(1):25–37.
27. Calì G, Timor-Trisch IE, Palacios-Jaraquemada J, et al. Changes in ultrasonography indicators of abnormally invasive placenta during pregnancy. Int J Gynaecol Obstet. 2018;140:319–25.
28. Calì G, Timor-Tritsch IE, Palacios-Jaraquemada J, et al. Outcome of cesarean scar pregnancy managed expectantly: systematic review and meta-analysis. Ultrasound Obstet Gynecol. 2018;51:169–75.
29. Timor-Tritsch IE, Monteagudo A, Cali G, et al. Cesarean scar pregnancy and early placenta accreta share common histology. Ultrasound Obstet Gynecol. 2014;43:383–95.
30. Ballas J, Pretorius D, Hull AD, Resnik R, Ramos GA. Identifying sonographic markers for placenta accreta in the first trimester. J Ultrasound Med. 2012;31(11):1835–41.
31. Cali G, Forlani F, Timor-Tritsch IE, et al. Natural history of Cesarean scar pregnancy on prenatal ultrasound: the crossover sign. Ultrasound Obstet Gynecol. 2017;50(1):100–4.
32. Shainker SA, Coleman B, Timor IE, Bhide A, Bromley B, Cahill AG, Gandhi M, Hecht JL, Johnson KM, Levine D, Mastrobattista J, Philips J, Platt LJ, Shamshirsaz AA, Shipp TD, Silver RM, Simpson LL, Copel JA, Abuhamad A. Society for Maternal-Fetal Medicine. Electronic

address: pubs@smfm.org. Special Report of the Society for Maternal-Fetal Medicine Placenta Accreta Spectrum Ultrasound Marker Task Force: consensus on definition of markers and approach to the ultrasound examination in pregnancies at risk for placenta accreta spectrum. Am J Obstet Gynecol. 2021;224(1):B2–B14.
33. Maynard H, Zamudio S, Jauniaux E, Collins SL. The importance of bladder volume in the ultrasound diagnosis of placenta accreta spectrum disorders. Int J Gynecol Obstet. 2018;140(3):332–7.
34. Bhide A, Sebire N, Abuhamad A, Acharya G, Silver R. Morbidly adherent placenta: the need for standardization. Ultrasound Obstet Gynecol. 2017;49:559–63.
35. Finberg HJ, Williams JW. Placenta accreta: prospective sonographic diagnosis in patients with placenta previa and prior cesarean section. J Ultrasound Med. 1992;11:333–43.
36. Collins SL, Ashcroft A, Braun T, et al. Proposal for standardized ultrasound descriptors of abnormally invasive placenta (AIP). Ultrasound Obstet Gynecol. 2016;47:271–5.
37. Jauniaux E, Collins S, Burton GJ. Placenta accreta spectrum: pathophysiology and evidence-based anatomy for prenatal ultrasound imaging. Am J Obstet Gynecol. 2018;218:75–87.
38. Zhang J, Li H, Wang F, Qin H, Qin Q. Prenatal diagnosis of abnormal invasive placenta by ultrasound: measurement of highest peak systolic velocity of subplacental blood flow. Ultrasound Med Biol. 2018;44(8):1672–8.
39. Shih JC, Palacios Jaraquemada JM, Su YN, et al. Role of three-dimensional power doppler in the antenatal diagnosis of placenta accreta: comparison with gray-scale and color doppler techniques. Ultrasound Obstet Gynecol. 2009;33(2):193–203.
40. Cali G, Giambanco L, Puccio G, Forlani F. Morbidly adherent placenta: evaluation of ultrasound diagnostic criteria and differentiation of placenta accreta from percreta. Ultrasound Obstet Gynecol. 2013;41(4):406–12.
41. Philips J, Gurganus M, DeShields S, et al. Prevalence of sonographic markers of placenta accreta spectrum in low-risk pregnancies. Am J Perinatol. 2019;36(8):733–80.
42. D'Antonio F, Iacovella C, Palacios-Jarquemada J, Bruno CH, Manzoli L, Bhide A. Prenatal identification of invasive placentation using magnetic resonance imaging :systematic review and meta-analysis. Ultrasound Obstet Gynecol. 2014;44:8–16.
43. Meng X, Xie L, Song W. Comparing the diagnostic value of ultrasound and magnetic resonance imaging for placenta accreta: a systematic review and meta-analysis. Ultrasound Med Biol. 2013;39(11):1958–65.
44. Palacios-Jaraquemada JM, Bruno CH, Martin E. MRI in the diagnosis and surgical management of abnormal placentation. Acta Obstet Gynecol Scand. 2013;92(4):392–7.
45. Dighe M. MR imaging of abnormal placentation. Magn Reson Imaging Clin N Am. 2017;25(3):601–10.
46. Maurea S, Romeo V, Mainenti PP, et al. Diagnostic accuracy of magnetic resonance imaging in assessing placental adhesion disorder in patients with placenta previa: correlation with histological findings. Eur J Radiol. 2018;106:77–84.
47. Chu C, Zhao S, Ding M, et al. Combining clinical characteristics and specific magnetic resonance imaging features to predict placenta accreta. J Comput Assist Tomogr. 2019;43(5):775–9.
48. Horowitz JM, Berggruen S, McCarthy RJ, et al. When timing is everything: are placental MRI examinations performed before 24 weeks' gestational age reliable? AJR Am J Roentgenol. 2015;205(3):685–92.
49. Patenaude Y, Pugash D, Lim K, et al. The use of magnetic resonance imaging in the obstetric patient. J Obstet Gynaecol Can. 2014;36(4):349–63.
50. Kanal E, Barkovich AJ, Bell C, et al. ACR guidance document on MR safe practices: 2013. J Magn Reson Imaging. 2013;37(3):501–30.
51. Salmanian B, Shamshirsaz A, Fox K, Meshinchi Asl N, Erfani H, Detlefs S, Coburn M, Espinoza J, Nassr A, Belfort M, Clark SL, Shamshirsaz AA. Clinical outcomes of a false positive antenatal diagnosis of placenta accreta spectrum. Am J Perinatol. 2021; Epub ahead of print

Chapter 7
Definitive Management of Placenta Accreta Spectrum

Pedro Viana Pinto, Ana Paula Machado, and Marina Moucho

Introduction

First reviewed by Irving and Hertig in 1937, the nomenclature of the placenta accreta spectrum (PAS) disorders has recently been endorsed by the International Federation of Gynaecology and Obstetrics (FIGO), including in its classification the abnormally adherent and invasive placenta [1, 2].

Peripartum hysterectomy, a surgical procedure often needed in the resolution of PAS, is defined by the World Health Organization as a maternal near-miss criterion. Traditionally, prevalence of peripartum hysterectomy in high-resource settings is relatively low. According to the literature, placental abnormalities (from placenta previa to PAS) are one of the principal causes of emergent postpartum hysterectomy, especially in high-income settings [3–5]. In a European study, prevalence of peripartum hysterectomy was 5.2 per 10,000 births ranging from 2.6 to 10.7 per 10,000 [6]. The most common indications were uterine atony (35.3%) followed by abnormally invasive placenta (34.8%) and uterine rupture (7.5%). Low and lower middle-income countries seem to have even higher prevalence [5].

Definitive management of the PAS disorders is considered in a majority of women, and even today, it is the preferred option in surveys conducted among members of the Society for Maternal-Fetal Medicine (SMFM) and FIGO expert panel [7, 8]. Caesarean hysterectomy is still regarded as the preferred treatment by the SMFM, Royal College of Obstetricians (RCOG) and Gynaecologists, FIGO and the International Society for Placenta Accreta Spectrum (IS-PAS), when preservation of

P. V. Pinto (✉)
Serviço de Ginecologia e Obstetrícia, Centro Hospitalar São João, Porto, Portugal

Faculdade de Medicina, Universidade do Porto, Porto, Portugal

A. P. Machado · M. Moucho
Serviço de Ginecologia e Obstetrícia, Centro Hospitalar São João, Porto, Portugal

S. A. Shazly, A. A. Nassr (eds.), *Placenta Accreta Spectrum*,
https://doi.org/10.1007/978-3-031-10347-6_7

fertility is not an issue [9–11]. It should be the preferred option especially in women with a PAS disorder with invasion of the parametrium or the uterine cervix, or women with an extensive invasion of the uterine wall by the placenta [10]. In a recent systematic review of 7001 cases of a PAS disorder, the pooled estimate for peripartum hysterectomy was 52.2% [12]. This procedure may be associated with high morbidity, ranging from postpartum haemorrhage to maternal death, including urinary tract, bowel or pelvic vessel injuries.

In this chapter, we discuss the definitive surgical management of PAS disorders, looking at preoperative planning and the surgical steps required to optimize outcomes.

Preoperative Preparation

The management of a PAS disorder involves careful preoperative planning and preparation to reduce the associated morbidity and mortality. Although the incidence of this pathology is growing, each centre may face the challenge of dealing with a limited number of cases, each one requiring an important level of expertise. The literature is consistent in defining the essential role of a multidisciplinary team in the management of PAS cases, and there is compelling evidence that after the introduction of a strict protocol with a multidisciplinary and experienced team, maternal and neonatal outcomes improve considerably, with women being less likely to require large volume blood transfusion, intensive care unit admission and reoperation within 7 days of delivery [13–20]. It is essential to understand that even in the best-case scenario, these patients must be considered as a real challenge. An obstetrician department with expertise in ultrasound and magnetic resonance imaging (MRI) of the placenta is essential for an accurate diagnosis, as there is evidence that an antenatal suspicion of a PAS disorder is associated with better maternal and foetal outcomes [21, 22]. Outcomes are also reportedly better in situations with planned delivery when comparing to emergent surgeries [21, 22]. It is essential to highlight the role of an experienced team, supporting the obstetric department: (a) anaesthesiology, with experience in approaching pregnant women and able to deal with situations of great haemodynamic instability and the need for massive blood transfusion; (b) gynaecological oncology, with skills in difficult pelvic surgery; (c) urology, to assist in cases of bladder involvement and reducing the risk of iatrogenic lesions of the urogenital tract; (d) the blood bank considering the high haemorrhagic risk, especially in cases with deep trophoblastic invasion, due to the eventual need for transfusion of blood derivatives and possible activation of a massive transfusion protocol; (e) interventional radiology for endovascular arterial occlusion in a situation of critical haemorrhage or for embolization of the uterine arteries; and (f) an intensive care unit prepared to receive critically ill patients. Also noteworthy are the roles of pathologists in the evaluation of hysterectomy specimens, essential to validate and clarify the diagnosis of a PAS disorder, and of neonatal intensive care units, considering that delivery is usually planned for the late preterm period. It may be reasonable to schedule early admission of the patient, in order to prepare the surgery and get all the support of the dedicated team and of the blood bank.

Late preterm delivery is recommended between 34 0/7 and 36 6/7 weeks of gestation [9–11]. A decision analysis indicates that delivery at 34 weeks of gestation may be optimal, balancing neonatal outcomes and the risk of maternal complications [23]. However, each case should be assessed individually, and it is adequate to adopt an expectant attitude until 36 weeks of gestation towards a pregnant woman with no vaginal bleeding or uterine contractions, no previous preterm birth or premature rupture of membranes and probably a more expeditious delivery in cases of women with some of these risk factors.

The decision to administer corticosteroids for induction of foetal lung maturity prior to delivery depends on each centre's local guidelines. While there is reasonable evidence for some benefits of its use in the late preterm group, there is still some controversy regarding its use [24, 25].

All patients should be screened for anaemia at the initial obstetric visit, and at any time of admission. The aim is to maintain a haematocrit above 30% with routine supplementation of iron and folic acid. Prevention of anaemia preoperatively is associated with decreased transfusion requirements. If anaemia is identified, a complete evaluation should be performed to adequately define its aetiology. It is essential to exclude iron deficiency and blood loss. Parenteral iron therapy is considered for those patients with iron deficiency anaemia who cannot tolerate or are noncompliant with oral therapy. Erythropoietin-stimulating agents and blood transfusions should be considered for patients with severe (haemoglobin <8 g/dL) or persistent anaemia.

Anaesthesia

Anaesthetic assessment preoperatively is essential. A thorough obstetric history should identify disorders that could affect intraoperative physiology and coagulation, including preeclampsia, thrombocytopenia and obstetric cholestasis, which may warrant further investigation. Previous anaesthetic experiences and difficulties should also be assessed. Preparation of surgery includes large-bore cannula (16G or 14G) and urinary catheter placement. The decision for general or regional anaesthesia should be shared with the patient and the multidisciplinary team. There is scarce evidence to favour one method over another. Regional anaesthesia confers some known advantages, from providing a more satisfactory maternal birth experience, minimizing uteroplacental drug transfer, avoiding airway manipulation and providing postoperative analgesia. Some studies reported less blood loss with regional anaesthesia compared with general anaesthesia in caesarean deliveries [26]. One potential drawback is the need for emergent conversion for general anaesthesia. In the event of epidural anaesthesia, it should be placed in the beginning of surgery, as it provides analgesia for other surgical steps (like ureteral stents or vascular catheterization). An induction of general anaesthesia would be the preferred option in cases where a difficult intubation is expected, where regional anaesthesia is contraindicated or when the patient states a preference. Also, in cases with antepartum bleeding, with higher risk of massive haemorrhage, it may also be the preferred option. Another choice is to perform a hybrid approach, with regional anaesthesia until baby delivery and general anaesthesia onwards. Ideally, it should be possible to induce anaesthesia, insert the artery balloon catheters and perform surgery in the same room.

Surgical Management of an Antenatally Suspected Case

Caesarean hysterectomy due to a PAS disorder may be particularly challenging, because of the abnormal vascularization with extensive collateral circulation and obliteration and distortion of the tissue planes, the possibility of partial organ resection and the potential for haemodynamic instability. Furthermore, this particularly defying surgery is even more difficult in the narrow space provided by the bony pelvis. Even in cases of placenta accreta or increta, there may exist distended and engorged vessels that could cause significant bleeding.

Preoperative planning is essential when placental abnormalities are suspected. Ultrasound and MRI images should be reviewed, and the possibility of bladder, cervical, parametrium or bowel invasion should be discussed. After adequate anaesthesia, consideration should be given to the placement of ureteral catheters. Cystotomy and ureteral injury are relatively common. Bladder injury may occur in approximately 7–48% of cases, and the rate of ureteral injury is around 2–6%, but may be as high as 18% [26]. According to a systematic review, placement of ureteral stents reduced the risk of lesion of these structures from 33% to 6%, during hysterectomy due to a PAS disorder [27]. The placement of ureteral stents may be especially useful in the presence of significant bleeding, making it easier to identify the ureters and prevent injury. Also, while placing the catheters, cystoscopy will allow the identification of signs of bladder mucosa invasion. Although a recent small retrospective cohort study concluded that ureteric stent placement did not reduce ureteral lesion during caesarean hysterectomy [28], the IS-PAS consensus opinion, even without a robust evidence, states that ureteric stents may be useful, especially in cases of placenta percreta, a recommendation similar to the one provided by the SMFM and FIGO [9–11, 26].

There is some controversy regarding the placement of balloon catheters in the pelvic vasculature, namely, in the internal or common iliac arteries or even the infrarenal aorta. This discussion is out of the scope of this chapter as it will be fully covered in another chapter of the book.

Regarding surgical incision, although there are no adequate comparative data as to which incision should be used, a vertical midline incision is typically performed, especially in cases of strong suspicion of a PAS disorder (Fig. 7.1a). It allows maximal exposure, facilitates an incision in cases of placenta percreta extending high up the uterine wall and allows exploration of the upper abdomen, pelvic sidewalls and retroperitoneum. Other options such the Maylard or Cherney incision, or a a curvilinear modified transverse incision (as proposed by Soleymani et al.) may also be considered.

It is essential to inspect the abdominal cavity and look for placental invasion of the bladder, bowel or parametria, as well as abdominal adhesions due to the

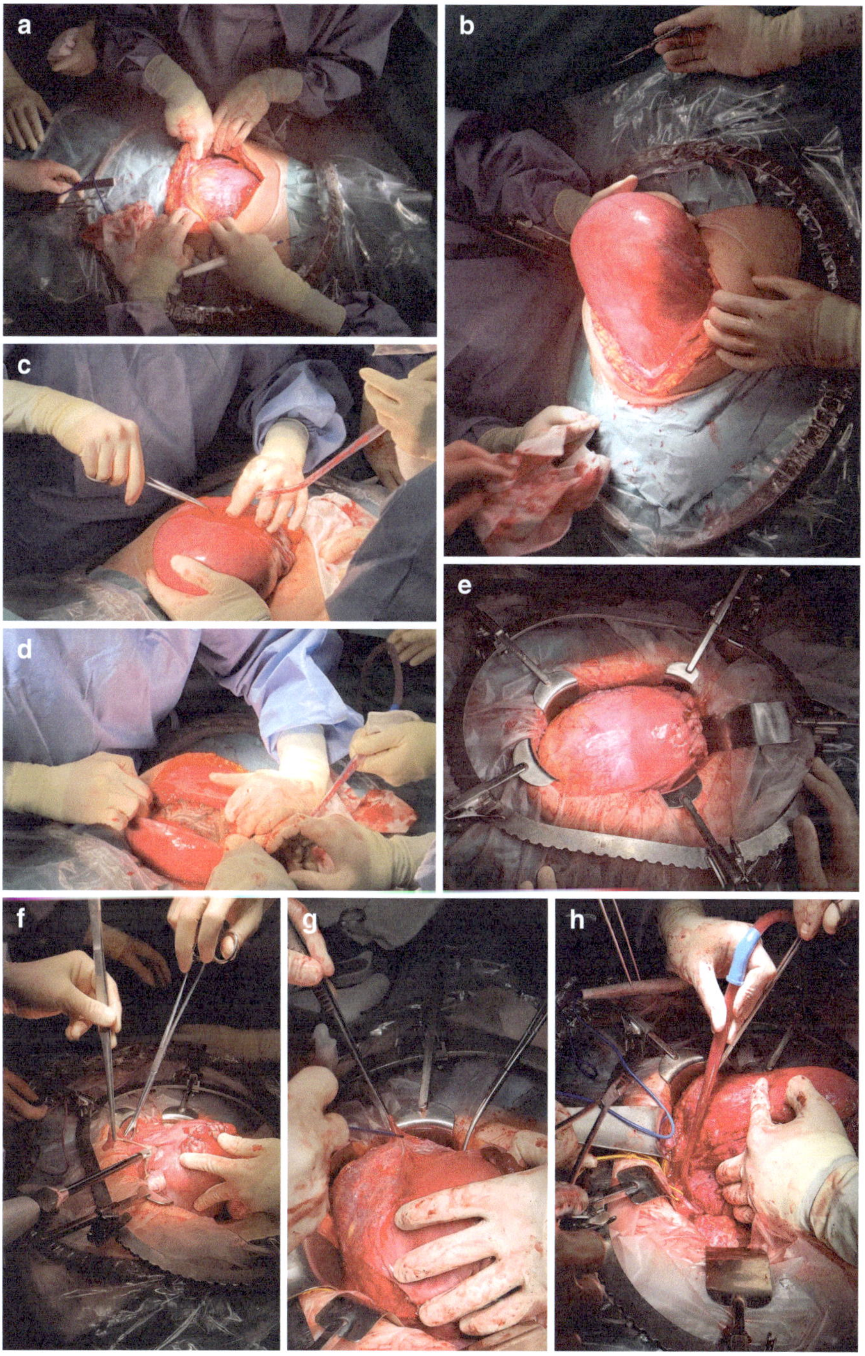

Fig. 7.1 (**a**) Midline vertical incision. (**b**) Uterine exposure and inspection of abdominal and pelvic cavities. (**c**, **d**) Uterine fundal incision for baby delivery. (**e**) Hysterotomy closure after umbilical cord clamping. (**f**) Opportunistic salpingectomy with a vessel sealing device. (**g**, **h**) Meticulous dissection of the vesico-uterine space; the uterus is pushed cephalad exposing the paravesical spaces, without disturbing the placental vasculature; the ureter is referenced in Figure **h**, making it safer and easier to complete this dissection

previous surgeries (Fig. 7.1b) Uterine incision should be high, avoiding the placental position (if necessary, intraoperative ultrasound may be performed). We suggest a fundal transverse incision (Figs. 7.1c–e), as reported by Matsubara et al., closing the incision after delivery of the baby [29]. If an antenatal diagnosis of a PAS disorder is uncertain, or if there is no clear invasion of the placenta into the uterus, it is reasonable to wait for spontaneous placental separation. In case of absence of placental separation, or gross placental invasion, it should be left in situ, the uterine incision closed and the hysterectomy performed. Attempts at forced placental removal often result in profuse haemorrhage and are strongly discouraged [9, 11, 26]. The use of uterotonics after the delivery of the baby will increase uterine contractility and may provide some separation of a partially adherent/invasive placenta, leading to increased blood loss. As a consequence, and following the IS-PAS and FIGO recommendations, uterotonics should not be used unless there is total placental separation and a PAS disorder is excluded [10, 26].

The recently published WOMAN Trial demonstrated that the administration of the antifibrinolytic, tranexamic acid, significantly reduced death due to obstetric haemorrhage when compared to placebo [30]. It is documented that its administration immediately after caesarean delivery significantly reduces intraoperative blood loss without significant side effects [26]. As a consequence, and although no studies specifically examined its efficacy in the management of a PAS disorder, its use seems justified in such high-risk surgery.

After the discovery of the tubal origin of some ovarian carcinomas (the tubal precursor lesion being the serous tubal intraepithelial carcinoma), it is adequate to perform opportunistic salpingectomy during hysterectomy without increasing the morbidity of the surgery. This recommendation, proven to be both safe and cost-effective, is supported by international guidelines [31–35]. These procedures may be performed either with simple suture and ligation or with a vessel sealing device (Fig. 7.1f). It is essential to avoid excessive upward traction on the uterus, which may cause significative bleeding.

Proceeding to the hysterectomy, it should be performed in the traditional way, starting by the division of the round ligaments. Once these procedures have been completed, it is important to gain wide access to the retroperitoneum and isolate the ureters; they should be easily identified if stents were placed previously. It may also be useful to isolate the internal iliac vessels and to identify the uterine artery at its origin. It can be easily accomplished at this point as, without any placental disruption, major blood loss is not expected.

Then, an approach should be made to the vesico-uterine space; access may be gained by a lateral or central approach, according to surgeon's preference and ease of access, and the bladder should be dissected away from the uterus until the bladder is at the anterior vaginal fornix level. This step may be very difficult, depending on the extension of invasion by the placenta. Meticulous dissection is crucial and intentional cystotomy may be necessary (Figs. 7.1g, h). This step is most commonly associated with important bleeding in cases with anterior placental invasion. Filling the bladder with a saline solution/methylene blue (either before or during surgery) may be important to help decrease surgical urological morbidity [29, 36–38]. It may be useful in helping to clearly identify the bladder top, avoiding inadequate dissection and making haemostasis easier. In cases of obvious bladder invasion, intentional cystotomy and cystectomy are easier and more feasible than trying to dissect the placenta away from the bladder [14, 38, 39]. Typically, this causes massive bleeding due to the engorged vessels, eventually ending up in cystectomy in the majority of cases, but with greater morbidity [26].

Continuing with the hysterectomy, the uterine arteries should be ligated as close to their origin from the anterior division of the internal iliac artery as possible. Dissection should be continued along the cardinal ligament until the uterus is freed to below the level of the placental attachment. After gaining access to the vagina, the uterus should be completely freed and removed. This is also a key moment in the surgery. It should be performed very carefully, especially in cases of cervical invasion that can make this a particularly challenging moment. Closing of the vaginal edge should be done in the traditional way and afterwards, haemostasis should be thoroughly reviewed. Some different surgical techniques have been proposed, mainly performed in a few cases, like a posterior uterine approach or the use of different sealing devices [40, 41].

Although scarce, the available evidence does not suggest that subtotal hysterectomy reduces morbidity and mortality when compared with total hysterectomy. The type of hysterectomy should be chosen according to the surgical team's experience and clinical scenario. In cases of a PAS disorder with cervical invasion, total hysterectomy should be the preferred treatment.

During surgery for a PAS disorder, the surgical team must be prepared to face abnormal bleeding, which may range from life-threatening to less severe. If tranexamic acid was not used previously, it may be reasonable to use its therapeutic dose in such cases. Although evidence is not strong enough to adequately conclude which is the best surgical method in cases of bleeding from a PAS disorder, there are some procedures that have been used. The internal iliac arteries may be ligated to decrease pelvic circulation, with conflicting results in the literature, but especially useful in situations where interventional radiology is not readily available; benefits are only temporary due to the extensive collateral vascularization during pregnancy [10, 38]; balloon occlusion of the internal iliac, common iliac or abdominal aorta has also been used with mixed results [42]; and vascular compression (mainly of the infra-renal aorta) can be used as a temporary measure to gain time until performing complete definitive treatment. Pelvic packing may be a life-saving measure in patients with uncontrollable haemorrhage; packing may be left in for 24 h to allow for optimization of clotting and haemostasis [10, 11].

There has been recent interest in the provision of a balanced transfusion regimen similar to that seen in the management of major trauma, aiming for a 1:1:1 ratio of packed red blood cells, plasma and platelets, especially in cases of a PAS surgery. Autologous cell salvage is an option to minimize allogenic red blood cell transfusion in select patients, such as those with high risk of massive obstetric haemorrhage, previous anaemia and rare blood types and/or those who refuse to take such products including Jehovah's witnesses [26]. Timely articulation with the blood bank is of extreme importance in case other clotting factors are needed, should a massive haemorrhage or a disseminated intravascular coagulopathy appear.

There is also conflicting evidence regarding delayed hysterectomy (leaving the placenta in the uterus at the time of delivery, with the intention of performing a hysterectomy later, in an attempt to reduce uterine perfusion) when compared to immediate hysterectomy [20, 43]. By allowing some resorption of the placenta, decrease in vascularity and involution of the uterus, defenders of this strategy argue that later surgery is easier. However, there is an associated risk of coagulopathy, haemorrhage and sepsis during the interim period. Patients should be alerted to these risks and need to be compliant with a rigorous follow-up, while the institution must be prepared for emergency hysterectomy and massive bleeding management. Delayed hysterectomies may be performed between 3 to 12 weeks postpartum [26]. Delaying hysterectomy in complex cases may reduce other surgical morbidity, especially in cases of a previously undiagnosed PAS disorder, with a surgical team without experience in managing these cases. In a systematic review of urinary tract injury rates with PAS disorders, there were no reported unintentional urological complications in nine cases of delayed hysterectomy; however, the sample size was too small to draw definitive conclusions. Intentional cystotomy and partial cystectomy were still required in one third of the cases [27]. Some cases of delayed hysterectomy performed by laparoscopy and even robotic surgery allow a better visualization of the surgical field with better haemostasis and enhanced recovery [44–46].

Lastly, it is important to consider some general recommendations:

(a) During surgery, the patient should be kept warm (either by patient warming devices or warmed intravenous infusions, or both). Inadvertent hypothermia causes inhibited platelet function, impaired coagulation and increased bleeding and is associated with an increased incidence of wound infection.
(b) Perioperative euvolaemia is also essential (avoiding excessive fluid infusion).
(c) Re-dosing of antibiotics in case of important blood loss or a prolonged surgery should also be considered.

Surgical Management of an Unexpected Case

In some situations, a PAS disorder may be obvious after entry into the abdomen, with the visualization of placental tissue at or beyond the uterine wall, extension into other pelvic organs or abnormal and highly exaggerated vascularization. It is essential to assess important active bleeding, the extent and location of placental invasion and the surgeon's expertise and available resources. In a stable situation (both foetal and maternal) without adequate clinical resources or expertise, it may be reasonable to close the abdominal wall and consider transfer to a reference centre; in a case with maternal stability but with foetal compromise, it may be possible to make a uterine incision remote from the placenta, deliver the baby and close the hysterotomy without disturbing the placenta and transfer the patient to a reference centre [9, 11]. If it is possible to gather an experienced team in time, it may also be possible to delay the uterine incision until there are adequate conditions to continue surgery.

In the case of an unstable patient, it is mandatory to proceed with surgery; fluid and blood resuscitation should be started as needed and infra-renal aortic compression may be a relatively simple technique that proves life-saving. It is also fundamental, at the same time, to bring together multidisciplinary team, including interventional radiology (if available), urology and the blood bank.

Postoperative Considerations

Depending on the length of surgery, blood loss and perioperative complications, the patient may need intensive haemodynamic monitoring, which can be provided in an intensive care unit. Patients should be closely monitored for blood loss, fluid overload, signs of infection and unnoticed complications (bowel, urinary). Clinical surveillance for any signs of organ failure is also important. Lastly, attention to the small but real possibility of Sheehan syndrome is warranted, given the clinical scenario.

Surgical Morbidity

Hysterectomy for a PAS disorder may be associated with important morbidity. As explained, blood loss is an important source of morbidity. A recent meta-analysis including data from over 7000 cases of PAS disorders reported a 46.9% incidence of haemorrhage requiring transfusion, with reports of a maximum volume loss of 20 L [12, 14, 47]. Coagulopathy is another serious morbidity that needs to be addressed and prevented aggressively. There are also several complications that may appear related to blood transfusions, ranging from a simple febrile reaction to circulatory overload with the risk of multiorgan failure. Infectious complications are rare nowadays. There are also specific complications associated with interventional radiology procedures, which are addressed in another chapter of this book. Bladder injuries are the most common intraoperative complication during surgery for a PAS disorder. Unintentional urinary tract injuries are described in 29% of caesarean hysterectomies, with 76% of these being bladder lacerations and 17%, ureteral injuries [27]. Major risk factors for urinary tract injury are the depth of placental invasion and intraoperative blood loss. Injury to other abdominal organs, such as the bowel, pelvic vessels and nerves, is rarer and also dependent on the extent of placental invasion and intraoperative haemorrhage.

Other intraoperative and perioperative complications include wound complications, reoperation, venous thromboembolism, pelvic abscess and prolonged hospital admission.

Very low mortality rates are possible in centres with expertise with these cases, essentially with antenatal diagnosis and multidisciplinary management [12]. Main risk factors for mortality are the depth of invasion, the availability of antenatal diagnosis and the presence of an experienced multidisciplinary team.

Psychological Impact

Postpartum hysterectomy due to a PAS disorder may be associated with a profound psychological impact. From the loss of fertility to the fear of death or other outcomes, women may be significantly affected by a diagnosis of a PAS disorder. Assessing psychological morbidity may be challenging in a condition like a PAS disorder. According to a small study reporting answers from 32 women submitted to surgery due to a PAS disorder, 70% of women indicated that diagnosis and treatment had created an emotional burden; 23.3% reported that establishing a bond with the newborn had been disturbed; and almost one third of the women reported the need for psychological support after surgery for a PAS disorder (half of the women submitted to caesarean hysterectomy) [48]. In another prospective study, using two validated survey tools, women with PAS at 36 months after surgery were more likely to report grief/depression and anxiety. During the majority of the study period, women were also more likely to report dyspareunia (around 50% of the study population). Regarding the quality of life evaluation, women with PAS reported lower scores in physical and social functioning domains at 36 months postpartum [49].

Situations of emergency postpartum hysterectomy show significant psychological impact, as well as sexual dysfunction [50]. As a consequence, the psychological impact of a caesarean hysterectomy for a PAS disorder is not unexpected. Practitioners should be aware and thoroughly investigate women's well-being after surgery and provide the adequate psychological support.

Conclusion

Caesarean hysterectomy is still the most widely performed treatment for a PAS disorder. It is clear that a multidisciplinary approach is associated with the best outcomes. Preoperative planning and a surgery performed by a team with adequate expertise is the key to preventing complications. With an adequate approach, blood loss and other surgical morbidities may be very much reduced.

References

1. Irving C, Hertig AT. A study of placenta accreta. Surg Gynecol Obstet. 1937;64:178–200.
2. Jauniaux E, Ayres-de-Campos D, Diagnosis FPA, Management Expert Consensus P. FIGO consensus guidelines on placenta accreta spectrum disorders: introduction. Int J Gynaecol Obstet. 2018;140(3):261–4.
3. de la Cruz CZ, Thompson EL, O'Rourke K, Nembhard WN. Cesarean section and the risk of emergency peripartum hysterectomy in high-income countries: a systematic review. Arch Gynecol Obstet. 2015;292(6):1201–15.
4. Maraschini A, Lega I, D'Aloja P, Buoncristiano M, Dell'Oro S, Donati S, et al. Women undergoing peripartum hysterectomy due to obstetric hemorrhage: a prospective population-based study. Acta Obstet Gynecol Scand. 2020;99(2):274–82.
5. van den Akker T, Brobbel C, Dekkers OM, Bloemenkamp KWM. Prevalence, indications, risk indicators, and outcomes of emergency peripartum hysterectomy worldwide: a systematic review and meta-analysis. Obstet Gynecol. 2016;128(6):1281–94.
6. Kallianidis AF, Maraschini A, Danis J, Colmorn LB, Deneux-Tharaux C, Donati S, et al. Epidemiological analysis of peripartum hysterectomy across nine European countries. Acta Obstet Gynecol Scand. 2020;99(10):1364–73.
7. Jolley JA, Nageotte MP, Wing DA, Shrivastava VK. Management of placenta accreta: a survey of maternal-fetal medicine practitioners. J Matern Fetal Neonatal Med. 2012;25(6):756–60.
8. Cal M, Ayres-de-Campos D, Jauniaux E. International survey of practices used in the diagnosis and management of placenta accreta spectrum disorders. Int J Gynaecol Obstet. 2018;140(3):307–11.
9. Jauniaux E, Alfirevic Z, Bhide AG, Belfort MA, Burton GJ, Collins SL, et al. Placenta praevia and placenta accreta: diagnosis and management: green-top guideline no. 27a. BJOG. 2019;126(1):e1–e48.
10. Collins SL, Alemdar B, van Beekhuizen HJ, Bertholdt C, Braun T, Calda P, et al. Evidence-based guidelines for the management of abnormally invasive placenta: recommendations from the International Society for Abnormally Invasive Placenta. Am J Obstet Gynecol. 2019;220(6):511–26.
11. Society of Gynecologic O, American College of O, Gynecologists, the Society for Maternal-Fetal M, Cahill AG, Beigi R, et al. Placenta accreta spectrum. Am J Obstet Gynecol. 2018;219(6):B2–B16.
12. Jauniaux E, Bunce C, Gronbeck L, Langhoff-Roos J. Prevalence and main outcomes of placenta accreta spectrum: a systematic review and meta-analysis. Am J Obstet Gynecol. 2019;221(3):208–18.
13. Shamshirsaz AA, Fox KA, Erfani H, Clark SL, Salmanian B, Baker BW, et al. Multidisciplinary team learning in the management of the morbidly adherent placenta: outcome improvements over time. Am J Obstet Gynecol. 2017;216(6):612. e1-e5
14. Shamshirsaz AA, Fox KA, Salmanian B, Diaz-Arrastia CR, Lee W, Baker BW, et al. Maternal morbidity in patients with morbidly adherent placenta treated with and without a standardized multidisciplinary approach. Am J Obstet Gynecol. 2015;212(2):218. e1-9
15. Fratto VM, Conturie CL, Ballas J, Pettit KE, Stephenson ML, Truong YN, et al. Assessing the multidisciplinary team approaches to placenta accreta spectrum across five institutions within the University of California fetal Consortium (UCfC). J Matern Fetal Neonatal Med. 2019:1–6.
16. Licon E, Matsuzaki S, Opara KN, Ng AJY, Bender NM, Grubbs BH, et al. Implementation of multidisciplinary practice change to improve outcomes for women with placenta accreta spectrum. Eur J Obstet Gynecol Reprod Biol. 2020;246:194–6.
17. Eller AG, Bennett MA, Sharshiner M, Masheter C, Soisson AP, Dodson M, et al. Maternal morbidity in cases of placenta accreta managed by a multidisciplinary care team compared with standard obstetric care. Obstet Gynecol. 2011;117(2 Pt 1):331–7.

18. Nieto AJ, Echavarria MP, Carvajal JA, Messa A, Burgos JM, Ordonez C, et al. Placenta accreta: importance of a multidisciplinary approach in the Colombian hospital setting. J Matern Fetal Neonatal Med. 2020;33(8):1321–9.
19. Smulian JC, Pascual AL, Hesham H, Qureshey E, Bijoy Thomas M, Depuy AM, et al. Invasive placental disease: the impact of a multi-disciplinary team approach to management. J Matern Fetal Neonatal Med. 2017;30(12):1423–7.
20. Schwickert A, van Beekhuizen HJ, Bertholdt C, Fox KA, Kayem G, Morel O, et al. Association of peripartum management and high maternal blood loss at cesarean delivery for placenta accreta spectrum (PAS): a multinational database study. Acta Obstet Gynecol Scand. 2021;
21. Warshak CR, Ramos GA, Eskander R, Benirschke K, Saenz CC, Kelly TF, et al. Effect of predelivery diagnosis in 99 consecutive cases of placenta accreta. Obstet Gynecol. 2010;115(1):65–9.
22. Eller AG, Porter TF, Soisson P, Silver RM. Optimal management strategies for placenta accreta. BJOG. 2009;116(5):648–54.
23. Robinson BK, Grobman WA. Effectiveness of timing strategies for delivery of individuals with placenta previa and accreta. Obstet Gynecol. 2010;116(4):835–42.
24. Gyamfi-Bannerman C, Thom EA, Blackwell SC, Tita AT, Reddy UM, Saade GR, et al. Antenatal betamethasone for women at risk for late preterm delivery. N Engl J Med. 2016;374(14):1311–20.
25. Saccone G, Berghella V. Antenatal corticosteroids for maturity of term or near term fetuses: systematic review and meta-analysis of randomized controlled trials. BMJ. 2016;355:i5044.
26. Allen L, Jauniaux E, Hobson S, Papillon-Smith J, Belfort MA, Diagnosis FPA, et al. FIGO consensus guidelines on placenta accreta spectrum disorders: nonconservative surgical management. Int J Gynaecol Obstet. 2018;140(3):281–90.
27. Tam Tam KB, Dozier J, Martin JN Jr. Approaches to reduce urinary tract injury during management of placenta accreta, increta, and percreta: a systematic review. J Matern Fetal Neonatal Med. 2012;25(4):329–34.
28. Crocetto F, Esposito R, Saccone G, Della Corte L, Sarno L, Morlando M, et al. Use of routine ureteral stents in cesarean hysterectomy for placenta accreta. J Matern Fetal Neonatal Med. 2021;34(3):386–9.
29. Matsubara S, Kuwata T, Usui R, Watanabe T, Izumi A, Ohkuchi A, et al. Important surgical measures and techniques at cesarean hysterectomy for placenta previa accreta. Acta Obstet Gynecol Scand. 2013;92(4):372–7.
30. Collaborators WT. Effect of early tranexamic acid administration on mortality, hysterectomy, and other morbidities in women with post-partum haemorrhage (WOMAN): an international, randomised, double-blind, placebo-controlled trial. Lancet. 2017;389(10084):2105–16.
31. Venkatesh KK, Clark LH, Stamilio DM. Cost-effectiveness of opportunistic salpingectomy vs tubal ligation at the time of cesarean delivery. Am J Obstet Gynecol. 2019;220(1):106. e1-e10
32. ACOG Committee opinion no. 774: opportunistic salpingectomy as a strategy for epithelial ovarian cancer prevention. Obstet Gynecol. 2019;133(4):e279–e84.
33. Salvador S, Scott S, Francis JA, Agrawal A, Giede C. No. 344-opportunistic salpingectomy and other methods of risk reduction for ovarian/fallopian tube/peritoneal cancer in the general population. J Obstet Gynaecol Can. 2017;39(6):480–93.
34. Ferrari F, Forte S, Prefumo F, Sartori E, Odicino F. Opportunistic salpingectomy during postpartum contraception procedures at elective and unscheduled cesarean delivery. Contraception. 2019;99(6):373–6.
35. Subramaniam A, Einerson BD, Blanchard CT, Erickson BK, Szychowski J, Leath CA 3rd, et al. The cost-effectiveness of opportunistic salpingectomy versus standard tubal ligation at the time of cesarean delivery for ovarian cancer risk reduction. Gynecol Oncol. 2019;152(1):127–32.
36. Celik S, Celik H, Soyer Caliskan C, Tosun M, Hatirnaz S. Bladder filling before accreta surgery is a very effective method for preventing bladder injury: a retrospective cohort study. J Matern Fetal Neonatal Med. 2019:1–6.

37. Pelosi MA 3rd, Pelosi MA. Modified cesarean hysterectomy for placenta previa percreta with bladder invasion: retrovesical lower uterine segment bypass. Obstet Gynecol. 1999;93(5 Pt 2):830–3.
38. Kingdom JC, Hobson SR, Murji A, Allen L, Windrim RC, Lockhart E, et al. Minimizing surgical blood loss at cesarean hysterectomy for placenta previa with evidence of placenta increta or placenta percreta: the state of play in 2020. Am J Obstet Gynecol. 2020;223(3):322–9.
39. Shamshirsaz AA, Fox KA, Erfani H, Belfort MA. The role of centers of excellence with multidisciplinary teams in the management of abnormal invasive placenta. Clin Obstet Gynecol. 2018;61(4):841–50.
40. Belfort MA, Shamshiraz AA, Fox K. Minimizing blood loss at cesarean-hysterectomy for placenta previa percreta. Am J Obstet Gynecol. 2017;216(1):78. e1-e2
41. Rossetti D, Vitale SG, Bogani G, Rapisarda AM, Gulino FA, Frigerio L. Usefulness of vessel-sealing devices for peripartum hysterectomy: a retrospective cohort study. Updat Surg. 2015;67(3):301–4.
42. Pinto PV, Machado AP, Montenegro N. Risk of hemorrhage in abnormally invasive placenta according to its management. J Matern Fetal Neonatal Med. 2017;30(18):2139–45.
43. Zuckerwise LC, Craig AM, Newton JM, Zhao S, Bennett KA, Crispens MA. Outcomes following a clinical algorithm allowing for delayed hysterectomy in the management of severe placenta accreta spectrum. Am J Obstet Gynecol. 2020;222(2):179. e1-e9
44. Skinner BD, Golichowski AM, Raff GJ. Laparoscopic-assisted vaginal hysterectomy in a patient with placenta percreta. JSLS. 2012;16(1):143–7.
45. Ochalski ME, Broach A, Lee T. Laparoscopic management of placenta percreta. J Minim Invasive Gynecol. 2010;17(1):128–30.
46. Rupley DM, Tergas AI, Palmerola KL, Burke WM. Robotically assisted delayed total laparoscopic hysterectomy for placenta percreta. Gynecol Oncol Rep. 2016;17:53–5.
47. van Beekhuizen HJ, Stefanovic V, Schwickert A, Henrich W, Fox KA, M MHG, et al. A multicenter observational survey of management strategies in 442 pregnancies with suspected placenta accreta spectrum. Acta Obstet Gynecol Scand. 2021;100:12.
48. Welz J, Keyver-Paik MD, Gembruch U, Merz WM. Self-reported physical, mental, and reproductive sequelae after treatment of abnormally invasive placenta: a single-center observational study. Arch Gynecol Obstet. 2019;300(1):95–101.
49. Grover B, Einerson BD, Keenan KD, Gibbins KJ, Callaway E, Lopez S, et al. Patient-reported health outcomes and quality of life after peripartum hysterectomy for placenta accreta spectrum. Am J Perinatol. 2020;39:281.
50. Fonseca A, Ayres de Campos D. Maternal morbidity and mortality due to placenta accreta spectrum disorders. Best Pract Res Clin Obstet Gynaecol. 2020;

Chapter 8
Conservative Management of Placenta Accreta Spectrum

Ismet Hortu, Elif Yagmur Erdem, and Ahmet Mete Ergenoglu

Definition

Placenta accreta spectrum (PAS) is a high-risk pregnancy condition resulting from abnormal adhesion of placental villi to myometrium. This spectrum, previously known as morbidly adherent placenta, includes different adhesion intervals: placenta accreta (trophoblasts are in contact with myometrium), placenta increta (trophoblasts invade myometrium), and placenta percreta (trophoblasts have passed the myometrium layer and in some cases cause invasion of adjacent tissue) [1, 2]. Although it is a newly defined term by FIGO, in association with increasing rates of cesarean delivery, today PAS is the most common reason for both hysterectomy associated with cesarean delivery and peripartum hysterectomy [3]. As it is a condition associated with high maternal morbidity and mortality rate, diagnosis and treatment of PAS is very important. The exact definition of the clinic of this condition before birth improves maternal and neonatal outcomes by ensuring patient's management by a multidisciplinary team with expertise.

Many hypotheses have been proposed to explain why and how PAS occur. The widely accepted hypothesis is that this process occurs with the iatrogenic defect at the endometrium-myometrial interface causing uncontrolled and excessive trophoblast invasion, loss of the normal structure of the decidua in the uterine scar area, abnormal vascularization, and secondary localized hypoxia [1].

I. Hortu (✉) · E. Y. Erdem · A. M. Ergenoglu
Department of Obstetrics and Gynecology, Ege University School of Medicine, Izmir, Turkey

S. A. Shazly, A. A. Nassr (eds.), *Placenta Accreta Spectrum*,
https://doi.org/10.1007/978-3-031-10347-6_8

Risk Factors

Although ultrasound is an indispensable evaluation in the diagnosis of PAS, the absence of ultrasound findings does not exclude the diagnosis. Therefore, clinical risk factors are equally important to ultrasound as a predictor of PAS [1]. Placenta previa is the most important risk factor for PAS and at one time was considered necessary for the diagnosis [4]. With placenta previa being the most important risk factor, the most common risk factor is previous cesarean delivery, which is responsible for the increase in the incidence of PAS [5]. Other risk factors include advanced maternal age, multiparity, and previous uterine surgery including endometrial curettage and assisted reproductive techniques [6], and with increased uterine conservation, previous retained placenta or placenta accreta has become a significant risk factor [4].

Clinical Presentation and Diagnosis

Antenatal diagnosis of the placenta accreta spectrum is very important and highly desirable because appropriate multidisciplinary clinical decisions can be made based on prenatal diagnosis, and potential maternal morbidity and mortality can be minimized with delivery in a level 3 maternal care facility [7]. Obstetric ultrasonography is the primary diagnostic modality for antenatal diagnosis with high specificity and sensitivity [8]. Women with relevant risk factors (e.g., one or more previous cesarean sections, placenta previa) should raise strong suspicion of PAS, and in this case, further investigation of the placental bed and ultrasound evaluation at the specialized center is required (Fig. 8.1) [9]. MRI can be of help if ultrasonography alone is inconclusive [10]. While clinical diagnosis can be made through inspection of the external surface of the uterus, confirmation can only be made after histopathological examination [11].

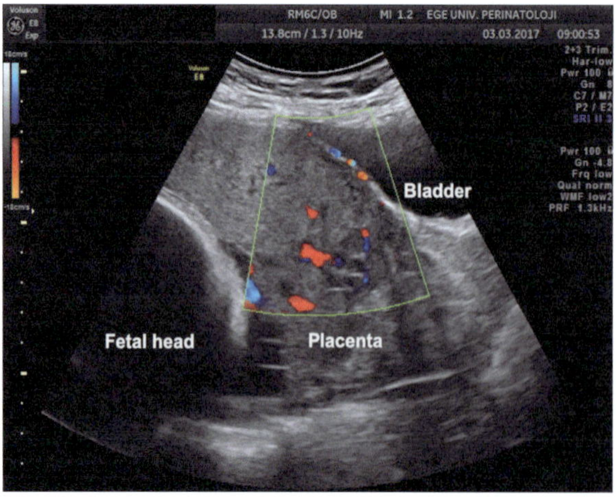

Fig. 8.1 Transabdominal sonographic view of placenta previa; color Doppler shows hypervascular placental bed

Management

Management of patients with PAS varies greatly based on personal experience, expert opinion, and clinical judgment. There are very few studies examining the management of PAS, and most of the information to guide the management are obtained from retrospective cohort studies and case series. Patients with suspected PAS should be informed about the diagnosis and all possible risks (e.g., blood transfusion, cesarean hysterectomy, need of maternal-fetal intensive care unit), and the patient's wishes should be taken into account in the management [12]. The main purpose in the management of PAS is to inform the patient (informed consent) and to develop a preoperative plan for the most appropriate intervention to reduce significant morbidity and potential mortality.

Timing of Delivery

Delivery should be planned when the necessary multidisciplinary team and facilities are provided in the most appropriate way. If there is no multidisciplinary team consisting of maternal-fetal medicine specialists, anesthesiologists, neonatologists, interventional radiologists, blood bank, nursing personnel, and support services at the place where the patient is planned to deliver, the patient should be transferred to the tertiary facility that has the capacity to manage possible major intraoperative bleeding in the most effective way and to provide postoperative maternal and fetal intensive care [12]. In a decision analysis to compare strategies for the timing of delivery in individuals with placenta previa and placenta accreta, planned delivery at 34 weeks of gestation resulted in the highest quality-adjusted life years under the base case assumptions [13]. In cases with a history of preterm labor, bleeding and contraction, or preterm premature rupture of membranes (PPROM), delivery can be provident before 34 weeks of gestation [3]. However, in asymptomatic placenta previa cases whose clinical and imaging findings indicate a low risk of PAS, delivery may be delayed until 35 or 36 weeks [3]. Delivery beyond 36 weeks of gestation is not recommended to avoid urgent delivery that may result in high morbidity and mortality, to prevent deeper invasion, and to allow conservative treatment planning [14]. In addition, considering that approximately half of women who are more than 36 weeks require urgent delivery for bleeding, the positive effects of the expected management on fetal maturation after this week of gestation decrease [12].

Cesarean Delivery and Hysterectomy

The most generally accepted approach to placenta accreta spectrum is planned cesarean hysterectomy [1]. The abdominal incision may be in the form of an infraumbilical midline incision or a Pfannenstiel. The choice between the two should be

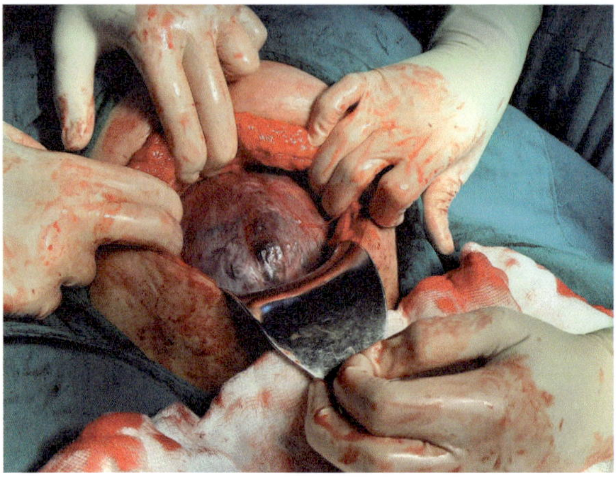

Fig. 8.2 Invasive placenta with increased vascularity that can be seen macroscopically during laparotomy

based on preoperative placental mapping by ultrasonography and operator's experience, and the uterine incision is done away from the placental bed and hysterectomy is initiated after fetal delivery [15]. Since there may be aberrant vessels in the ureterovesical junction in PAS cases, not defining the bladder borders properly and making an erroneous high incision can cause risky consequences such as vascular damage and severe bleeding (Fig. 8.2) [15]. By inserting a preoperative three-way Foley catheter and filling the bladder with methylene blue during surgery, the border of the bladder is determined, and it is aimed to reduce the risk of urological injury [15].

Hysterectomy is also not considered a risk-free approach. It has some disadvantages include bladder or bowel injury, fistulas, and massive bleeding, which may occur as the abnormal invasive placenta can receive the blood supply from the vessels originating from the upper segment of the vagina [11]. Collaboration with the blood bank is very important, as the risk of bleeding is high during this approach and large volume blood transfusion may be required [15]. Besides the physical loss of the uterus due to hysterectomy, there are also psychological negative effects. Since the uterus is associated with fertility and femininity by many women, women perceive hysterectomy as a loss of female identity [10, 16].

Conservative Management

Conservative approaches in the treatment of PAS include strategies aimed at avoiding hysterectomy, preserving fertility, as well as reducing maternal morbidity and mortality [15]. Conservative management includes four different methods: (1) extirpative treatment, (2) leaving placenta in situ known as expectant management, (3) one-step conservative surgery, and (4) Triple P procedure [17].

I. *Extirpative treatment*: This is a procedure in which the placenta is manually removed during surgery [18]. The main purpose of this approach is not to leave the placental tissue in the uterus, which is seen as one of the first steps in managing postpartum hemorrhage, and at the same time to preserve the uterus [19]. However, most surgeons specializing in the management of PAS disorders consider that attempts at manual removal of the placenta should be avoided as forced removal of the placenta will be associated with massive hemorrhagic bleeding [20].

II. *Leaving the placenta in situ*: In this approach, also called expectant management, umbilical cord ligated close to its placental insertion after delivery of the baby, the hysterotomy is closed in the standard fashion with leaving the placenta in situ without any attempt to remove the placenta [20]. The main purpose of this method, which is firstly applied in cases with hysterectomy cesarean section with high complication risk, is to avoid morbidities associated with hysterectomy such as massive hemorrhage and to preserve fertility [17]. By leaving the placenta in situ, the placenta is progressively and spontaneously separated from the uterus secondary to decreased blood circulation in the uterus and necrosis of villous tissue [19]. Since the placenta remains in the uterus, complications such as infection, coagulation disorders, and even fistula, peritonitis, uterine necrosis, and septic shock may occur later [8]. Adjunctive procedures such as the use of methotrexate, prophylactic uterine artery embolization, and hysteroscopic resection of retained tissues have been proposed to hasten placental resorption and reduce these complications [17]. The time to a spontaneous resolution ranges from 4 weeks to 9–12 months, with a mean of 6 months [20].

II a. *Gentle attempted removal of the placenta*: It is possible to remove the "non-accreta" placental part in cases of PAS disorders visibly limited to a small part of the uterine wall, or false-positive PAS cases without clinical evidence, where bleeding can be stopped with compression sutures [20]. However, because of the risk of massive obstetric bleeding and the need for urgent hysterectomy, a multidisciplinary team should be available and ready [19].

II b. *Methotrexate adjuvant treatment*: Compared to early pregnancy period, the low rate of trophoblast cell cycle decreases the effectiveness of methotrexate in the late period. In addition, side effects such as neutropenia and medullary aplasia due to methotrexate use increase the occurrence of complications such as secondary infection that may occur due to the placenta being left in situ [17]. The only case of maternal death reported after conservative treatment was attributed to the development of myelosuppression, nephrotoxicity, and septic shock due to the application of methotrexate into the umbilical cord [18].

II c. *Hysteroscopic resection of retained placental tissue*: In a retrospective multicenter study conducted by Sentilhes et al., involving 167 women and 131 of whom had successful conservative treatments, hysteroscopic resection or curettage or both were used to remove the retained placenta in 29 (25%) cases, at median of 20 weeks (range 2–45 weeks) after delivery [18]. In a series of 23 women with PAS who received conservative treatment in which the placenta is left in situ, 12 patients with retained placenta tissue had persistent bleeding or pelvic pain and undergo hysteroscopic procedures [21]. Complete resection was achieved in 5 of these 12 patients after the first procedure, 2 patients after the second procedure, and 4 patients after the third procedure, but 1 patient required hysterectomy due to persistent bleeding and anemia after the first procedure [21].

II d. *Prophylactic uterine embolization:* Such techniques as stepwise uterine surgical devascularization, bilateral uterine or hypogastric artery surgical ligation, iliac artery embolization, or balloon occlusion are performed together with interventional radiology in prophylaxis and active treatment of bleeding during the conservative treatment of PAS [19]. With these interventions, the surgeon can reduce intraoperative blood loss, prevent secondary bleeding with prophylactic development, and increase the rate of placental resorption [19]. However, this technique is also associated with significant maternal morbidity; major complications include puncture site hematoma, femoral arterial pseudoaneurysm, vascular damage, thromboembolic events, abscess, uterine necrosis, leg ischemia, and ischemic injury to the femoral nerve [15]. Larger studies are needed to demonstrate the safety and efficacy of these adjuvant techniques in the treatment of PAS disorders.

III. *One-step conservative surgery:* This procedure aims to reduce bleeding and restore the uterine anatomy to minimize recurrence of PAS in the next pregnancy [8]. One-step conservative surgery was first described in 2004 by Palacios et al. In a series of 68 cases with anterior placenta percreta [22], applied electively in 49 patients and urgently in 19 patients, this technique allowed resection of the invasive myometrium when 50% or less of the anterior uterine circumference was involved. Hemostasis was achieved with selective vascular ligation, brace or box sutures, and fibrin glue. After the excision, myometrial defect, myometrial suture, fibrin glue, and polyglycolic mesh were repaired. The uterus was preserved in 50 (74%) of 68 women, and hysterectomy was required in 18 cases (26%). Of the hysterectomies, 16 were indicated for massive destruction and two were helpful for coagulopathies. Of the 42 cases, ten became pregnant and these pregnancies resulted in an uncomplicated cesarean section. The following surgical complications have occurred in the cases: pelvic bleeding (one), coagulopathies (two), uterine infection (three), low ureteral ligations (two), iatrogenic foreign bodies (two), and collection (three). In conclusion, this approach may not be suitable in patients with extensive invasion, but it has allowed an adequate uterine repair in cases of anterior placenta percreta with a defined area of focal involvement. This technique can also be advantageous for low- and middle-income countries where it is not possible to access expensive additional treatments such as interventional radiology [16, 19].

IV. *Triple P procedure:* This procedure aims to reduce the morbidity associated with PAS hysterectomy [8]. The Triple P procedure, first described by Chandraharan et al., constitutes three main steps: (1) perioperative determination of the superior border of the placenta by transabdominal ultrasonography, (2) preoperative placement of intra-arterial balloon catheters and pelvic devascularization, and (3) no attempt to remove the entire placenta with large myometrial excision and uterine repair [11]. Interventional radiology plays a role in the realization of this technique in which hemostasis is achieved by placing prophylactic occlusive balloons in the internal iliac to reduce vascularity feeding the placental bed before myometrial excision [11]. During excision, the 2 cm myometrium border is preserved above the bladder edge to allow the myometrial defect to close and bleeding from the separated and adherent part of the placenta is controlled by oversewing the defect [17]. When the posterior bladder wall is involved, placental tissue invading the bladder is left in situ to avoid cystotomy or further dissection [20].

Follow-Up After Conservative Management

Although there is not sufficient information about the length of the follow-up period, the patient is observed in the hospital for 8 days when the risk of bleeding and infection is the highest [17]. Antibiotic prophylaxis is applied for 5 days during this follow-up. Since there is still a risk of bleeding and infection, the patient and her partner are informed about the need for long-term follow-up before discharge. The patient should be advised about emergencies such as hyperthermia, severe pelvic pain, malodorous vaginal discharge, and excessive bleeding. The patient should be called for a weekly visit during the first 2 months, and clinical evaluation, pelvic ultrasound, and laboratory screen for infection should be performed during the visit [15].

Long-Term Considerations

The risk of recurrence of PAS depends on the procedure used in the treatment performed and the number of treatments. Following the conservative treatment of PAS, there is a risk of uterine synechiae and amenorrhea, and the risk of uterine rupture is predicted in pregnancies following the treatment [20]. Although a limited number of successful pregnancy cases have been reported, more data are needed on this subject.

References

1. Cahill AG, Beigi R, Heine RP, Silver RM, Wax JR. Placenta Accreta Spectrum. Am J Obstet Gynecol. 2018;219(6):B2–B16. https://doi.org/10.1016/j.ajog.2018.09.042.
2. Shazly SA, Hortu I, Shih J, Melekoglu R, Fan S, Ahmed F, Karaman E, Fatkullin I, Pinto PV, Irianti S, Tochie JN, Abdelbadie AS, Salah MA, Abd Elazeem HAS, Saad MM, Ergenoglu

AM, Yeniel AO, Sagol S, Itil IM, et al. Prediction of success of uterus preserving management in women with placenta accreta spectrum (CON-PAS score): A multicenter international study. Int J Gynaecol Obstet. 2020;2020:1–8. https://doi.org/10.1002/ijgo.13518.
3. Silver RM, Branch DW. Placenta Accreta Spectrum. N Engl J Med. 2018;378(16):1529–36. https://doi.org/10.1056/nejmcp1709324.
4. Carusi DA. The placenta accreta spectrum: epidemiology and risk factors. Clin Obstet Gynecol. 2018;61(4):733–42. https://doi.org/10.1097/GRF.0000000000000391.
5. Silver RM, Landon MB, Rouse DJ, Leveno KJ, Spong CY, Thom EA, Moawad AH, Caritis SN. Repeat cesarean deliveries. Acog. 2006;107(6):1226–32.
6. Jauniaux E, Grønbeck L, Bunce C, Langhoff-Roos J, Collins SL. Epidemiology of placenta previa accreta: a systematic review and meta-analysis. BMJ Open. 2019;9(11):1–9. https://doi.org/10.1136/bmjopen-2019-031193.
7. Committee R, No O. Obstetric care consensus no. 7: placenta Accreta spectrum. Obstet Gynecol. 2018;132(6):E259–75. https://doi.org/10.1097/AOG.0000000000002983.
8. Palacios-Jaraquemada JM. Conservative vs. radical management of Placenta Accreta Spectrum (PAS). Curr Obstet Gynecol Rep. 2020;9(1):36–43. https://doi.org/10.1007/s13669-019-00274-9.
9. Morlando M, Collins S. Placenta accreta spectrum disorders: challenges, risks, and management strategies. Int J Women's Health. 2020;12:1033–45. https://doi.org/10.2147/IJWH.S224191.
10. Palacios-Jaraquemada JM, Fiorillo A, Hamer J, Martínez M, Bruno C. Placenta accreta spectrum: a hysterectomy can be prevented in almost 80% of cases using a resective-reconstructive technique. J Matern Fetal Neonatal Med. 2020;0(0):1–8. https://doi.org/10.1080/14767058.2020.1716715.
11. Piñas Carrillo A, Chandraharan E. Placenta accreta spectrum: risk factors, diagnosis and management with special reference to the triple P procedure. Womens Health. 2019;15 https://doi.org/10.1177/1745506519878081.
12. Silver RM, Levine D. Management of the placenta accreta spectrum (placenta accreta, increta, and percreta); 2018. p. 1–13.
13. Robinson BK, Grobman WA. Effectiveness of timing strategies for delivery of individuals with placenta previa and accreta. Obstet Gynecol Surv. 2011;66(1):4–6. https://doi.org/10.1097/OGX.0b013e3182021db5.
14. El-Agwany AS. Conservative surgical management of placenta accreta: partial myometrial excision techniques. Eur J Obstet Gynecol Reprod Biol. 2021;256(xxxx):521–2. https://doi.org/10.1016/j.ejogrb.2020.11.017.
15. Sichitiu J, El-Tani Z, Mathevet P, Desseauve D. Conservative surgical management of placenta Accreta spectrum: a pragmatic approach. J Investig Surg. 2019;0(0):1–9. https://doi.org/10.1080/08941939.2019.1623956.
16. Karaman E, Kolusarı A, Çetin O, Çim N, Alkış I, Yıldızhan R, Şahin HG, Gül A. Local resection may be a strong alternative to cesarean hysterectomy in conservative surgical management of placenta percreta: experiences from a tertiary hospital, J Matern Fetal Neonatal Med. 2017;30(8):947–52. https://doi.org/10.1080/14767058.2016.1192119.
17. Sentilhes L, Kayem G, Silver RM. Conservative management of placenta accreta spectrum. Clin Obstet Gynecol. 2018b;61(4):783–94. https://doi.org/10.1097/GRF.0000000000000395.
18. Kayem G, Provansal M, Perrotin F, Winer N, Pierre F, Benachi A, Dreyfus M, Bauville E, Mahieu-caputo D, Descamps P, Bretelle F. Treatment of placenta Accreta. Obstet Gynecol. 2010;115(3):526–34.
19. Sentilhes L, Kayem G, Chandraharan E, Palacios-Jaraquemada J, Jauniaux E, Duncombe G, Klaritsch P, Chantraine F, Kingdom J, Grønbeck L, Rull K, Nigatu B, Tikkanen M, Sentilhes L, Asatiani T, Leung WC, AlhaidariT, Brennan D, Kondoh E, et al. FIGO consensus guidelines on placenta accreta spectrum disorders: conservative management. Int J Gynecol Obstet. 2018a;140(3):291–8. https://doi.org/10.1002/ijgo.12410.

20. Fox KA, Shamshirsaz AA, Carusi D, Secord AA, Lee P, Turan OM, Huls C, Abuhamad A, Simhan H, Barton J, Wright J, Silver R, Belfort MA. Conservative management of morbidly adherent placenta: expert review. Am J Obstet Gynecol. 2015;213(6):755–60. https://doi.org/10.1016/j.ajog.2015.04.034.
21. Legendre G, Zoulovits FJ, Kinn J, Senthiles L, Fernandez H. Conservative Management of Placenta Accreta: Hysteroscopic resection of retained tissues. J Minim Invasive Gynecol. 2014;21(5):910–3. https://doi.org/10.1016/j.jmig.2014.04.004.
22. Palacios Jaraquemada JM, Pesaresi M, Nassif JC, Hermosid S. Anterior placenta percreta: surgical approach, hemostasis and uterine repair. Acta Obstet Gynecol Scand. 2004;83(8):738–44. https://doi.org/10.1111/j.0001-6349.2004.00517.x.

Chapter 9
Adjunctive Treatment of Placenta Accreta Spectrum

Sohum C. Shah, Karin A. Fox, and Ahmed A. Nassr

Introduction

In this chapter, we provide an overview about therapies that may offer benefit in conjunction with cesarean hysterectomy, which is the most common and definitive treatment of the placenta accreta spectrum (PAS). We also discuss techniques used as adjunctive therapies with conservative and uterine sparing management, which may be applied perioperatively. Specifically, we discuss the interventional modalities that focus on preventing maternal hemorrhage. This includes vascular embolization, prophylactic arterial balloon occlusion, and use of the antifibrinolytic agent tranexamic acid. We also briefly discuss the controversy surrounding methotrexate and why its use is not recommended, and the investigational technique of high-intensity focused ultrasound (HIFU).

Surgical Control of Bleeding

There are several different techniques that have been described for bleeding control in cases of PAS which include intra-arterial embolization, intra-arterial balloon occlusion, arterial ligation, intrauterine tamponade, and the use of uterine compression sutures.

S. C. Shah · K. A. Fox · A. A. Nassr (✉)
Department of Obstetrics and Gynecology, Baylor College of Medicine and Texas Children's Hospital, Houston, TX, USA
e-mail: Ahmed.Nassr@bcm.edu

S. A. Shazly, A. A. Nassr (eds.), *Placenta Accreta Spectrum*,
https://doi.org/10.1007/978-3-031-10347-6_9

Uterine Artery Embolization

Uterine artery embolization (UAE) is a procedure most commonly used to treat symptomatic fibroids [1]. Other indications include postpartum hemorrhage, inoperable gynecologic tumors, and occlusion of uterine vascular malformations [2]. The procedure is contraindicated in the setting of suspected gynecologic malignancies, ongoing gynecologic infection, and ongoing pregnancy [3]. In the case of life-threatening hemorrhage, UAE may be performed regardless of the clinical scenario, when the benefits outweigh the risks [4]. The procedure is performed by interventional radiologists. The embolic materials most commonly used for uterine or vaginal hemorrhage are Gelfoam slurry, pledgets, coils, or n-butyl-2-cyanoacrylate, whereas particles such as tris-acryl gelatin microspheres or polyvinyl alcohol are used for embolization of fibroids. The procedure is performed by first gaining vascular access via the common femoral or the radial artery, and passing a guidewire to the intended target. Angiogram is performed to map the arterial tree and to locate the uterine arteries. The ipsilateral anterior oblique view allows for optimal visualization of the uterine artery. A 4- or 5-Fr catheter or a larger lumen microcatheter is placed at the transverse portion of the uterine artery, distal to the cervicovaginal branches, to prevent unintentional embolization of other arteries [5]. The goal of treatment is to slow blood flow within the uterine artery and thus decrease uterine perfusion pressure, rather than to cause complete occlusion of the artery. The most common complications of uterine artery embolization are amenorrhea and persistent vaginal discharge [6]. However, given the indication for UAE in the case of PAS, when hysterectomy is planned and performed, these complications become less significant.

Arterial embolization as a treatment for postpartum hemorrhage in cases of PAS is supported by evidence-based data [7]. It can be used as an adjunctive therapy with conservative management or with hysterectomy. In a systematic review of 177 pregnant patients who had pelvic arterial embolization in the setting of conservative management, secondary hysterectomy was avoided in 90% of patients [8]. It has been available as a highly successful treatment modality for postpartum hemorrhage for years [7]. However, arterial embolization for PAS differs significantly from cases of postpartum hemorrhage due to uterine atony. The chaotic periuterine hypervascularization between the bladder and lower uterine segment in PAS is predominantly venous in nature; therefore, arterial embolization does not directly occlude these vessels. Additionally, periuterine fibrosis makes surgical dissection challenging, no matter where the vessels are located. Bugling placental tissue may increase the difficulty in mapping or easily accessing target arteries. Other arteries that may be involved in the uteroplacental vasculature are the ovarian, pudendal, obturator, sacral, and inferior epigastric arteries. Embolizing these aberrant vessels could inadvertently cause ischemic events in organs such as the bladder or bowel [9].

Most reports focus on using arterial embolization in conjunction with conservative management. In one retrospective study, median estimated blood loss (EBL), transfusion requirements, and length of intensive care unit (ICU) stay were compared between a UAE group that underwent UAE following delivery and prior to hysterectomy and a control group who received only cesarean hysterectomy. There was a significant difference in EBL (P = 0.04), 1500 (range 500–2000) vs 2000 (range 1000–4500), respectively. There was not a significant difference in length of ICU stay or transfusion requirements. In a subgroup analysis, women with placenta increta had a significant decrease in length of ICU stay (P = 0.04) and transfusion requirements (P = 0.009). Thus, the authors concluded that for placenta increta, UAE following cesarean delivery and prior to hysterectomy appears to be safe and effective in decreasing blood loss, transfusion requirements, and length of ICU stay compared with cesarean hysterectomy alone [10]. Other studies have described UAE prior to cesarean delivery; however, this poses the risks of exposing the fetus to radiation, and decreasing oxygen supply to the fetus, causing the surgeons to rush in attempts to decrease time from embolization to delivery [11, 12].

Internal Iliac Artery Ligation

Direct ligation of the internal iliac artery has been described, specifically several retrospective studies studying outcomes in women who had this procedure performed at the time of delivery. However, in one study, with the strength of having a comparative group (patients who did not undergo internal iliac artery ligation), the authors' conclusion could not corroborate a reduction in blood loss. In this study, patients with PAS who did and did not receive intraoperative internal iliac artery ligation were analyzed for blood loss and length of hospitalization. Among 23 cases, there was neither a significant difference in blood loss nor length of hospital stay [13]. Notably, patients who did not have cesarean hysterectomy for management were excluded from this study. A subsequent randomized controlled trial confirmed the lack of difference of estimated intraoperative blood loss in patients with PAS who underwent cesarean hysterectomy between groups who had internal iliac artery ligation and those who did not. Additionally, the group who underwent internal iliac artery ligation had significantly longer operative time [14].

Although internal iliac artery ligation is conventionally accepted as an effective means to control blood loss intraoperatively, with studies showing up to 49% reduction in pelvic blood flow and 85% reduction in pulse pressure, cesarean hysterectomy in the context of PAS presents additional challenges [13, 15]. The time needed to achieve adequate hemostasis, presence of collateral vessels, and excess blood flow from other vessels (external iliac, inferior epigastric, inferior mesenteric arteries) and potential occlusion of the operative field by lateral placental extension are all contributory factors [13]. Additionally, experience in identification of the internal iliac artery and appropriate ligation is necessary to avoid ligation and occlusion of more proximal vessels.

Endovascular Balloon Occlusion of the Pelvic Circulation

Endovascular balloon occlusion of the pelvic circulation is another strategy that has been increasingly attempted as an adjunct intraoperative strategy [7]. The procedure can be done in several ways, including occlusion of the internal iliac arteries (PBOIIA), common iliac arteries (PBOCIA), abdominal aorta (PBOAA), and uterine arteries (PBOUA). It can be performed in conjunction with or in lieu of UAE. Of these, aortic balloon occlusion has been shown to be associated most consistently with the reduced blood loss. Conversely, balloon occlusion of the internal iliac and common iliac arteries has been shown to result in higher lower-limb complications such as claudication and thrombosis [16].

One systematic review found a statistically significant difference in blood loss for cesarean section and cesarean hysterectomy in pregnancies complicated by PAS (−310 mL, $P = 0.020$) with use of PBOIIA compared to no endovascular intervention [16]. Additionally, the authors found reduced amount of packed red blood cells transfused in all patients who underwent endovascular occlusion compared to those who did not during delivery (−1.54 units of packed red blood cells, $P = 0.001$). Operative time and length of hospital stay were not significantly different. There were, however, significant complications that arose from endovascular balloon occlusion including bladder injury, ureteral injury, disseminated intravascular coagulopathy (DIC), vesicovaginal and vesicouterine fistula formation, rebleeding requiring further intervention, lower limb claudication, arterial thrombosis, balloon rupture, access vessel pseudoaneurysm, and groin hematoma [16]. Based on this systematic review and another small randomized controlled trial, the International Society for Placenta Accreta Spectrum (IS-PAS) does not recommend routine use of prophylactic pelvic arterial balloon catheters (Grade B recommendation) [7].

Uterine Compression Sutures

Uterine compression sutures include methods such as B-Lynch, Hayman, Pereira, Cho, and other techniques [17–21]. Several studies have reported the use of compression sutures in conjunction with uterine artery ligation, intrauterine balloon tamponade, and focal resection for uterine preservation in PAS cases [22–28]. In a large case series, 26 women had bilateral uterine artery ligation performed, followed by placement of a B-Lynch suture—compression achieved by suturing the anterior and posterior uterine walls together [23]. B-Lynch suture is well described as a treatment for uterine atony. The ligation was first performed with a simple stitch, using 1.0 chromic suture. B-Lynch was then performed, followed by double-layer closure of the hysterotomy. Although this technique was effective in preserving fertility in cases of atony and bleeding from placental remnants, the limitations and drawbacks were noted. Placenta accreta spectrum and DIC were proposed as reasons for failure of the B-Lynch procedure. Although bleeding from atony was well controlled by the B-Lynch suture, there likely needs to be additional steps to control bleeding from the placental bed [23]. It is difficult to comment about the use compression sutures independently, as it was used in conjunction with arterial ligation or other measures in most of the studies described above.

Use of Tranexamic Acid

The WOMAN trial was a large, multicenter, double-blinded, placebo-controlled randomized controlled trial that compared tranexamic acid (TXA) to placebo to prevent death from all causes of peripartum bleeding [29]. 20,021 gravidae were included in the primary analysis, and there were 483 maternal deaths, in which 72% of these deaths were attributed to bleeding. The study concluded that the risk ratio due to bleeding for patients who received 1 gram of TXA within 3 h of delivery was 0.78 ($P = 0.03$). In the WOMAN trial, if bleeding continued after 30 min of first administration of TXA or stopped and restarted within 24 h, 1 gram of TXA was re-dosed [29]. The risk reduction with regard to all causes of mortality was not statistically significant. Importantly, the risk of thromboembolic events did not differ between the groups, nor did the rate of sepsis [29]. The CRASH-2 trial, a study of trauma patients, came to the same conclusion; however, this study demonstrated reduction in all-cause mortality [30]. While neither of these studies was specific to treatment of the PAS, given that PAS results in increased blood loss compared to cesarean or vaginal delivery absent PAS, and that massive transfusion is often required, it is plausible that early administration of TXA is reasonable when anticipating massive transfusion. One international PAS database study analyzed factors associated with severe postpartum hemorrhage defined as either estimated blood loss >3500 mL or ≥ 5500 mL (the 75th and 95th percentiles for the cohort). Neither prophylactic nor therapeutic tranexamic acid use correlated with a difference in blood loss; however, the authors concluded that the lack of difference with therapeutic use was due to the indication for ongoing bleeding rather than lack of efficacy [31]. This relatively inexpensive, low-risk intervention still may be considered in patients with PAS and future, well-designed trials are needed [7].

With regard to uterotonic agents and procoagulant agents, there is not enough data validating their use directly related to PAS. Therefore, IS-PAS recommends using uterotonic agents in compliance with local policies. Hemostatic agents and procoagulant agents should be used at the discretion of the surgeon (class D evidence) [7].

Investigational Therapies

High-Intensity Focused Ultrasound

High-intensity focused ultrasound (HIFU) is another modality that has been proposed for the management of PAS. HIFU is a noninvasive treatment that results in thermal damage directly to a targeted area without an effect on the surrounding tissue. It has been used historically in the management of solid tumors [32] and more recently has been used for treatment of uterine leiomyomas, cesarean scar pregnancies, and adenomyosis [33, 34]. A recently published systematic review of four articles highlighted its potential application to PAS as an adjunct to conservative management [35].

One study included patients who had vaginal deliveries with retained PAS only [36], whereas the three remaining studies included patients who had either cesarean delivery or vaginal delivery [37–39]. The studies had strict inclusion criteria, which included exclusion of patients with active postpartum hemorrhage, extensive abdominal scarring, and genital infection. Additionally, all studies included combined treatment with uterine curettage or hysteroscopic resection, and methotrexate in selected cases. For the one study in which only vaginal deliveries were included, inclusion criteria included patients with (1) stable vital signs without active bleeding or infection, (2) normal liver and renal function, (3) hemoglobin greater than 7, (4) residual placenta area greater than or equal to 3 cm by 3 cm but covering less than half the uterine cavity, (5) desire to preserve fertility and breastfeed, (6) declining surgery and chemical therapy, and (7) no prior conservative approach before HIFU therapy [36]. Generally, the procedure is safe, with a low incidence of complications (less than 1%), and highly effective for women who strongly desire uterine preservation. However, the limitations of this procedure are noticeable.

In all included studies, a HIFU system was used for the procedure. This included an ultrasound transducer with a generator (to produce the therapeutic energy), a diagnostic ultrasound imaging device, a movement system controlled by a computer to drive the transducer, a specialized treatment bed, and a degassed water circulation unit. The procedure was performed with the patient lying in the prone position, allowing the lower abdomen to be in contact with degassed water. The location, size, and shape of the residual placenta, along with adjacent organs, were then mapped out with assistance of the ultrasound-based computer system. The residual placental tissue was divided into slices of 5 mm in width, and each slice was ablated in 5-second bursts, from deepest to most superficial point of infiltration. Ultrasound scans were performed before and after the treatment, to ensure that the target area was captured [36].

The number of patients with PAS who may be eligible for HIFU is severely limited by the requisite strict selection criteria—patients with PAS may have significant adhesive disease, and are at greater risk for significant hemorrhage, and definitive management should not be delayed. Patients who are hemodynamically stable with active bleeding are generally eligible for endovascular occlusion procedures;

however, this is not the case for HIFU. There is a need for more evidence-based data to further understand the role of HIFU in PAS prior to widespread adoption.

Methotrexate

Methotrexate therapy has been suggested as an adjuvant therapy for the conservative management of placenta accreta spectrum and is highly controversial [40]. In a systematic review which studied conservative management strategies, there were 17 patients who received methotrexate. Six percent of these patients required a delayed hysterectomy despite treatment. There were no deaths reported in the methotrexate group in this study [41]; however, the route of administration of methotrexate was not specified. In a retrospective study performed in China, 54 women with confirmed placenta increta who desired conservative management received either systemic methotrexate intravenously or local multipoint injection under ultrasound guidance. The treatment was considered successful if hysterectomy was avoided. In the systemic group, which included 21 patients, 4 underwent hysterectomy for uncontrollable postpartum hemorrhage and infection. In the local administration group, which included 33 patients, 8 patients needed dilation and curettage as placenta was not delivered spontaneously. However, there were no instances of hysterectomy in this subgroup. There were no maternal deaths in the study [42]. In a larger French multicenter study, there were 167 patients included who were treated with conservative management including methotrexate. There was one maternal death attributed to methotrexate therapy, when it was injected into the umbilical cord [43].

Methotrexate works by disrupting the folic acid pathway in rapidly dividing cells such as first and second trimester trophoblasts. Trophoblasts' division is limited and does not appear to contribute significantly to placental growth in the later stages of pregnancy; therefore, there is no biologic plausibility for the mechanism of action of methotrexate, and it likely does not reduce the volume of the placenta [44]. Methotrexate is immunosuppressive, which can be harmful in the case of PAS, as patients are already at higher risk of morbidity due to longer operative time—the risk for infection and sepsis may be therefore be exacerbated with methotrexate therapy. Methotrexate can cause pancytopenia, nephrotoxicity, and toxic accumulation when injected intra-umbilically [41]. Based on these risks, the IS-PAS consensus guidelines strongly recommend against using methotrexate [7].

Conclusions

Many adjunctive treatments may be used singly or in combination in addition to the gold standard treatment for PAS—hysterectomy. These strategies can also be used in conjunction with conservative management. Emerging strategies need further investigation and may provide a wider array of novel options for PAS management.

References

1. Ravina J, Ciraru-Vigneron N, Bouret J, Herbreteau D, Houdart E, Aymard A, et al. Arterial embolisation to treat uterine myomata. Lancet. 1995;346(8976):671–2.
2. Vedantham S, Goodwin SC, McLucas B, Mohr G. Uterine artery embolization: an underused method of controlling pelvic hemorrhage. Am J Obstet Gynecol. 1997;176(4):938–48.
3. Momah-Ukeh I, Ertreo M. Uterine artery embolization. Essential interventional radiology review. Springer; 2022. p. 567–77.
4. Pelage J-P, Le Dref O, Mateo J, Soyer P, Jacob D, Kardache M, et al. Life-threatening primary postpartum hemorrhage: treatment with emergency selective arterial embolization. Radiology. 1998;208(2):359–62.
5. Salazar GM, Petrozza JC, Walker TG. Transcatheter endovascular techniques for management of obstetrical and gynecologic emergencies. Tech Vasc Interv Radiol. 2009;12(2):139–47.
6. Varghese K, Adhyapak S. Therapeutic Embolization. Springer; 2017.
7. Collins SL, Alemdar B, van Beekhuizen HJ, Bertholdt C, Braun T, Calda P, et al. Evidence-based guidelines for the management of abnormally invasive placenta: recommendations from the International Society for Abnormally Invasive Placenta. Am J Obstet Gynecol. 2019;220(6):511–26.
8. Mei J, Wang Y, Zou B, Hou Y, Ma T, Chen M, et al. Systematic review of uterus-preserving treatment modalities for abnormally invasive placenta. J Obstet Gynaecol. 2015;35(8):777–82.
9. Pan Y, Zhou X, Yang Z, Cui S, De W, Sun L. Retrospective cohort study of prophylactic intra-operative uterine artery embolization for abnormally invasive placenta. Int J Gynecol Obstet. 2017;137(1):45–50.
10. Wang M, Ballah D, Wade A, Taylor AG, Rizzuto G, Li B, et al. Uterine artery embolization following cesarean delivery but prior to hysterectomy in the management of patients with invasive placenta. J Vasc Interv Radiol. 2019;30(5):687–91.
11. Niola R, Giurazza F, Nazzaro G, Silvestre M, Nasti G, Di Pasquale MA, et al. Uterine artery embolization before delivery to prevent postpartum hemorrhage. J Vasc Interv Radiol. 2016;27(3):376–82.
12. Matsubara S. Re: uterine artery embolization before delivery to prevent postpartum hemorrhage. J Vasc Interv Radiol. 2016;27(7):1101–2.
13. Iwata A, Murayama Y, Itakura A, Baba K, Seki H, Takeda S. Limitations of internal iliac artery ligation for the reduction of intraoperative hemorrhage during cesarean hysterectomy in cases of placenta previa accreta. J Obstet Gynaecol Res. 2010;36(2):254–9.
14. Hussein AM, Dakhly DMR, Raslan AN, Kamel A, Abdel Hafeez A, Moussa M, et al. The role of prophylactic internal iliac artery ligation in abnormally invasive placenta undergoing caesarean hysterectomy: a randomized control trial. J Matern Fetal Neonatal Med. 2019;32(20):3386–92.
15. Camuzcuoglu H, Toy H, Vural M, Yildiz F, Aydın H. Internal iliac artery ligation for severe postpartum hemorrhage and severe hemorrhage after postpartum hysterectomy. J Obstet Gynaecol Res. 2010;36(3):538–43.
16. Shahin Y, Pang CL. Endovascular interventional modalities for haemorrhage control in abnormal placental implantation deliveries: a systematic review and meta-analysis. Eur Radiol. 2018;28(7):2713–26.
17. B-Lynch C, Coker A, Lawal AH, Abu J, Cowen MJ. The B-Lynch surgical technique for the control of massive postpartum haemorrhage: an alternative to hysterectomy? Five cases reported. BJOG Int J Obstet Gynaecol. 1997;104(3):372–5.
18. Pereira A, Nunes F, Pedroso S, Saraiva J, Retto H, Meirinho M. Compressive uterine sutures to treat postpartum bleeding secondary to uterine atony. Obstet Gynecol. 2005;106(3):569–72.
19. Hayman R, Arulkumaran S, Steer P. Uterine compression sutures: surgical management of postpartum hemorrhage. Obstet Gynecol. 2002;99(3):502–6.
20. Cho JH, Jun HS, Lee CN. Hemostatic suturing technique for uterine bleeding during cesarean delivery, vol. 96. Elsevier; 2000. p. 129.

21. Takahashi H, Baba Y, Usui R, Suzuki H, Horie K, Yano H, et al. Matsubara–Yano suture: a simple uterine compression suture for postpartum hemorrhage during cesarean section. Arch Gynecol Obstet. 2019;299(1):113–21.
22. Shazly SAE, Badee AY, Ali MK. The use of multiple 8 compression suturing as a novel procedure to preserve fertility in patients with placenta accreta: case series. Aust N Z J Obstet Gynaecol. 2012;52(4):395–9.
23. Shahin AY, Farghaly TA, Mohamed SA, Shokry M, Abd-El-Aal D-EM, Youssef MA. Bilateral uterine artery ligation plus B-Lynch procedure for atonic postpartum hemorrhage with placenta accreta. Int J Gynecol Obstet. 2010;108(3):187–90.
24. Mohamed MA, Mohammed AH. Parallel vertical compression sutures to control bleeding in cases of placenta previa and accreta. J Matern Fetal Neonatal Med. 2019;32(4):641–5.
25. Zhu L, Lu J, Huang W, Zhao J, Li M, Zhuang H, et al. A modified suture technique for the treatment of patients with pernicious placenta previa and placenta accreta spectrum: a case series. Ann Trans Med. 2021;9(14):1140.
26. ElNoury MAH, Webster SN, Abdelhalim DA. ElNoury–Webster bundle: a preemptive surgical approach with a modified lower B-Lynch compression suture to manage morbidly low or adherent placenta. J Matern Fetal Neonatal Med. 2021:1–4.
27. Ratiu AC, Crisan DC. A prospective evaluation and management of different types of placenta praevia using parallel vertical compression suture to preserve uterus. Medicine. 2018;97(46):e13253.
28. Shih JC, Liu KL, Kang J, Yang JH, Lin MW, Yu CU. 'Nausicaa' compression suture: a simple and effective alternative to hysterectomy in placenta accreta spectrum and other causes of severe postpartum haemorrhage. BJOG Int J Obstet Gynaecol. 2019;126(3):412–7.
29. Shakur H, Roberts I, Fawole B, Chaudhri R, El-Sheikh M, Akintan A, et al. Effect of early tranexamic acid administration on mortality, hysterectomy, and other morbidities in women with post-partum haemorrhage (WOMAN): an international, randomised, double-blind, placebo-controlled trial. Lancet. 2017;389(10084):2105–16.
30. Shakur H, Roberts I, Bautista R, Caballero J, Coats T, Dewan Y, et al. Effects of tranexamic acid on death, vascular occlusive events, and blood transfusion in trauma patients with significant haemorrhage (CRASH-2): a randomised, placebo-controlled trial. Lancet. 2010;376(9734):23.
31. Schwickert A, van Beekhuizen HJ, Bertholdt C, Fox KA, Kayem G, Morel O, et al. Association of peripartum management and high maternal blood loss at cesarean delivery for placenta accreta spectrum (PAS): a multinational database study. Acta Obstet Gynecol Scand. 2021;100:29–40.
32. Orsi F, Arnone P, Chen W, Zhang L. High intensity focused ultrasound ablation: a new therapeutic option for solid tumors. J Cancer Res Ther. 2010;6(4):414.
33. Jeng C-J, Ou K-Y, Long C-Y, Chuang L, Ker C-R. 500 cases of high-intensity focused ultrasound (HIFU) ablated uterine fibroids and adenomyosis. Taiwanese J Obstet Gynecol. 2020;59(6):865–71.
34. Hong Y, Guo Q, Pu Y, Lu D, Hu M. Outcome of high-intensity focused ultrasound and uterine artery embolization in the treatment and management of cesarean scar pregnancy: A retrospective study. Medicine. 2017;96(30):e7687.
35. Abd Elazeem HAS, Saad MM, Ahmed IA, Sayed EG, AlMahdy AM, Atef F, et al. High-intensity focused ultrasound in management of placenta accreta spectrum: A systematic review. Int J Gynecol Obstet. 2020;151(3):325–32.
36. Bai Y, Luo X, Li Q, Yin N, Fu X, Zhang H, et al. High-intensity focused ultrasound treatment of placenta accreta after vaginal delivery: a preliminary study. Ultrasound Obstet Gynecol. 2016;47(4):492–8.
37. Ye M, Yin Z, Xue M, Deng X. High-intensity focused ultrasound combined with hysteroscopic resection for the treatment of placenta accreta. BJOG Int J Obstet Gynaecol. 2017;124:71–7.
38. Jiang X, Tang Q, Yang B, Ye F, Cai L, Wang X, et al. High-intensity focused ultrasound combined procedures treatment of retained placenta accreta with marked vascularity after abortion or delivery. Int J Hyperth. 2019;36(1):420–6.

39. Liu Y, Zhang WW, He M, Gong C, Xie B, Wen X, et al. Adverse effect analysis of high-intensity focused ultrasound in the treatment of benign uterine diseases. Int J Hyperth. 2018;35(1):56–61.
40. Arulkumaran S, Ng C, Ingemarsson I, Ratnam S. Medical treatment of placenta accreta with methotrexate. Acta Obstet Gynecol Scand. 1986;65(3):285–6.
41. Steins Bisschop CN, Schaap TP, Vogelvang TE, Scholten PC. Invasive placentation and uterus preserving treatment modalities: a systematic review. Arch Gynecol Obstet. 2011;284(2):491–502.
42. Zhang C, Li H, Zuo C, Wang X. Retrospective analysis: conservative treatment of placenta increta with methotrexate. J Obstet Gynaecol Res. 2018;44(5):907–13.
43. Sentilhes L, Ambroselli C, Kayem G, Provansal M, Fernandez H, Perrotin F, et al. Maternal outcome after conservative treatment of placenta accreta. Obstet Gynecol. 2010;115(3):526–34.
44. Khan M, Sachdeva P, Arora R, Bhasin S. Conservative management of morbidly adherant placenta–a case report and review of literature. Placenta. 2013;34(10):963–6.

Chapter 10
Prediction and Risk Reduction of Clinical Outcomes of Placenta Accreta Spectrum

Mohamed I. Ateya, Ahmed S. Sedik, Islam A. Ahmed, Mostafa H. Abouzeid, and Sherif A. Shazly

Introduction

Placenta accreta spectrum (PAS), previously termed adherent or invasive placental disorder, is a major obstetric condition that may lead to detrimental maternal outcomes [1, 2]. The magnitude of PAS has been substantially potentiated in the current century in response to the rising trend of cesarean deliveries worldwide [3]. Therefore, PAS has no longer become a rare incidence, and obstetricians'/gynecologic surgeons' exposure to PAS management experience has expended over time. Although the rising rate of PAS cases has been overwhelming to obstetric practice and health systems, it has enhanced our understanding of these disorders and encouraged extensive research to promote early diagnosis and facilitate evidence-based clinical decisions [4].

In the last few decades, our understanding of PAS has considerably developed, including our awareness of PAS risk factors [5]. Recognition of risk factors, accompanied by emerging imaging expertise, has led to robust strategies of antenatal characterization and early diagnosis of PAS [6]. More recently, evolving clinical studies proposed risk stratification systems of women with presumed diagnosis of PAS to predict their peripartum outcomes and contribute to counseling, decision-making, and management planning [7].

M. I. Ateya
Department of Obstetrics and Gynecology, South Valley University, Qena, Egypt

A. S. Sedik · I. A. Ahmed
Faculty of Medicine, Assiut University, Assiut, Egypt

M. H. Abouzeid
Women Health Hospital, Assiut University, Assiut, Egypt

S. A. Shazly (✉)
Department of Obstetrics and Gynecology, Leeds Teaching Hospitals NHS Trust, Leeds, UK
e-mail: sherif.shazly@nhs.net

S. A. Shazly, A. A. Nassr (eds.), *Placenta Accreta Spectrum*,
https://doi.org/10.1007/978-3-031-10347-6_10

In this chapter, we will primarily focus on clinical predictors of clinical outcomes in women with presumed PAS during pregnancy, with special emphasis on their role in risk stratification and management decision prior to delivery.

PAR-A (Placenta Accreta Risk–Antepartum) and PAR-P (Placenta Accreta Risk–Peripartum) Scores

Score Development

PAR-A and PAR-P scores were introduced to the literature in 2020 [7]. The scores were originally developed using an international database, which was created for the purpose of that study. The database comprises antenatal, peripartum, and postpartum data of 727 women, recruited from 11 tertiary centers, with presumed PAS, which was confirmed at birth. The two scores were created using machine learning algorithms and were tested internally using a testing subset of the data [7].

Score Components

Both scores were designed to predict significant morbidity in women with PAS, primarily PAS-associated massive blood loss (≥ 2500 mL). Other predicted outcomes include maternal admission to intensive care unit (ICU) after birth and prolonged postpartum hospitalization. PAR-A score considers antenatally determined factors only in predicting these outcomes. Therefore, the score can be calculated shortly after diagnosis is suspected in order to stratify maternal risk of significant adverse maternal outcomes. The most contributing factors to PAR-A score are number of previous cesarean deliveries, Asian ethnicity, parity, centrally situated placentas, and prenatal hemoglobin level (Fig. 10.1). PAR-P score combines both antenatal and intrapartum factors to predict the same outcomes. Unlike PAR-A score which serves as a tool for risk stratification and counseling, PAR-P score enables testing of different management scenarios of the same patient in priori to predict clinical outcomes. Accordingly, PAR-P score may be used to decide an individualized management plan and endorse alternative strategies based on intraoperative findings prior to delivery. Diagnostic modality, parametrial invasion, intrapartum diagnosis of PAS, bladder invasion, and uterine incision away from placental site yield the highest impact on PAR-P score (Fig. 10.2) [7].

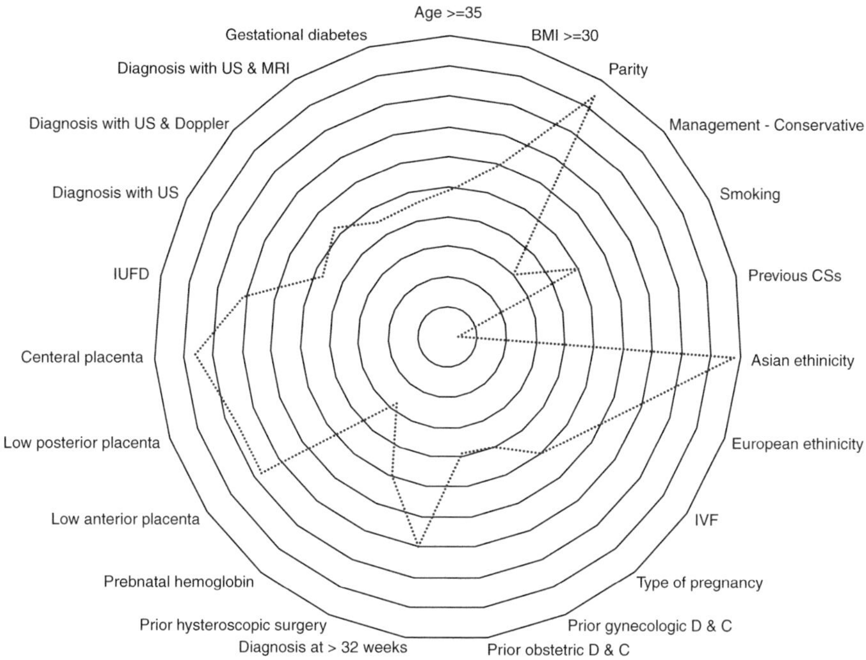

Fig. 10.1 Magnitude of contribution of antepartum characteristics to PAR-A score. * *BMI* body mass index, *CS* cesarean section, *IVF* in vitro fertilization, *D&C* dilation and curettage, *IUFD* intrauterine fetal death, *US* ultrasound, *MRI* magnetic resonance imaging

Score Performance

In the primary study, PAR-A score predicted PAS-associated massive blood loss, prolonged hospitalization, and admission to ICU with an area under curve (AUC) of 0.84, 0.81, and 0.82, respectively [7]. Recently, PAR-A score was externally validated through a prospective multicenter study, that was conducted by six PAS-specialized centers. Results were comparable to the original study; AUC of PAS-associated massive blood loss was 0.85 (95% confidence interval [CI] 0.74–0.95), and 0.88 (95% CI 0.81–0.95) for ICU admission [8]. PAR-P score yielded AUC of 0.86, 0.90, and 0.86 for PAS-associated massive blood loss, prolonged hospitalization, and admission to ICU, respectively, as reported by the original study [7].

Score Applicability

Unlike traditional statistics, machine learning-based scores are complex and do not rely on straight, and fully interpretable calculations. Therefore, clinical implementation of these scores requires software applications that run the algorithm of the

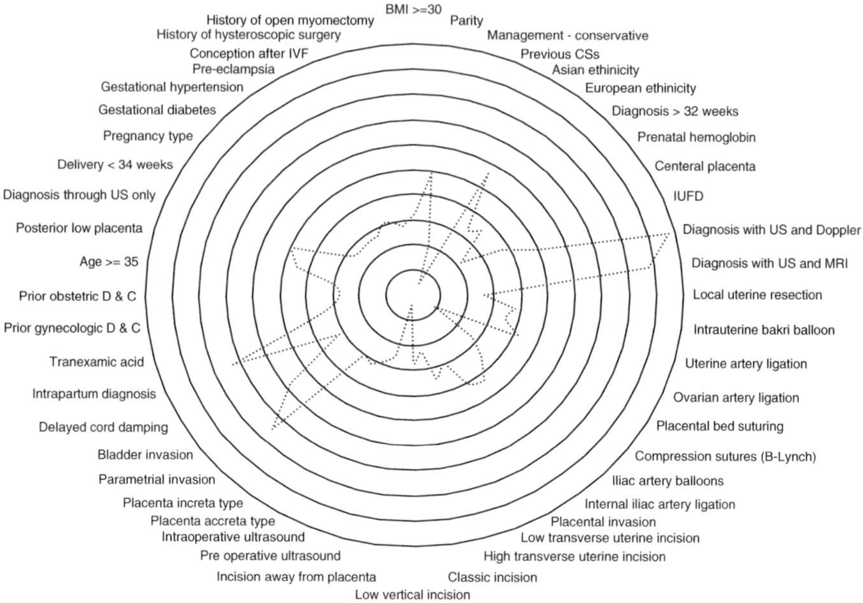

Fig. 10.2 Magnitude of contribution of antepartum characteristics to PAR-P score. * *BMI* body mass index, *CS* cesarean section, *IVF* in vitro fertilization, *D&C* dilation and curettage, *IUFD* intrauterine fetal death, *US* ultrasound, *MRI* magnetic resonance imaging

created model and produce a final result. A tool was developed by SilverAxon® (SilverAxon For artificial intelligence-based medical software, Egypt), in collaboration with PAR score research team [9]. Patient and disease features are provided through the software interface to calculate the output, which presents as a score from 1 to 12 depending on probability, sensitivity, and specificity of prediction of adverse outcomes, i.e., massive blood loss and admission to ICU, and is plotted on the corresponding area receiver operating characteristic (ROC) curve (Fig. 10.3).

Interpretation of the score should be made carefully since it focuses primarily on sensitivity and specificity. According to basic statistical understanding, sensitivity indicates high score ability to recognize women who would develop the outcome (complications). In other words, high sensitivity of, e.g., massive blood loss indicates that the risk of this complication is unlikely missed and that most women developing the complication are recognized. Similarly, low sensitivity conveys that many patients who would develop massive blood loss are likely not diagnosed. On the other hand, high specificity denotes that development of the complication is highly likely, while low specificity means that most diagnosed patients are not actually at risk [10]. In practice, clinicians should cautiously consider whether they would prioritize high sensitivity, high specificity, or a balanced point of both depending on the nature of the condition. Sensitivity may be superior to specificity in serious and life-threatening conditions since the score should miss as few cases as possible, while specificity may be superior when overdiagnosis could be associated

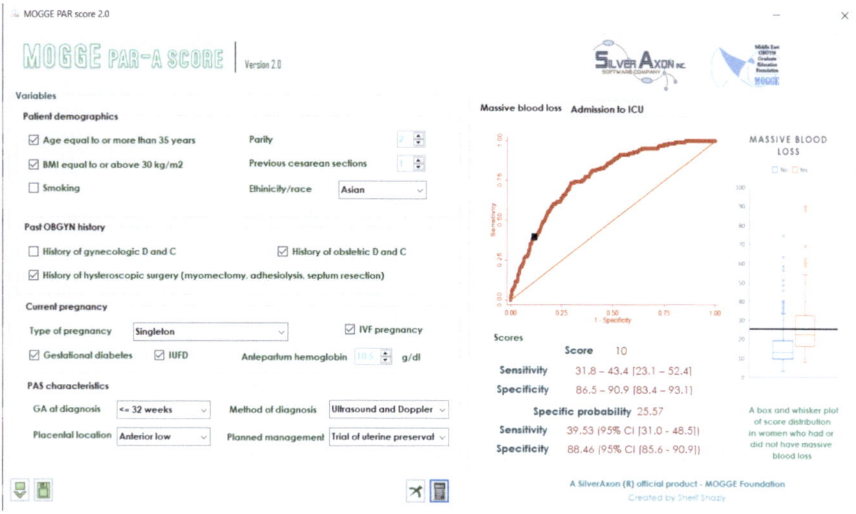

Fig. 10.3 PAR-A score calculator

with significant sequences such as unnecessary interventions or high costs. In PAS patients, both parameters are important. Nevertheless, sensitivity is more critical. Overall, this information may assist risk stratification, which subsequently supports decision-making on managing facility, preparation for delivery, decision for hospitalization, and possible need for additional measures, e.g., interventional radiology.

Disadvantages and Limitations

Since these scores were developed using retrospective databases, they acquire the same inherent limitations of these studies. Specifically, retrospective studies reveal associations between variables and the outcome, which do not necessarily indicate causality. For example, administration of tranexamic acid slightly contributes to worse outcomes according to PAR-P score [7] while clinically, administration of tranexamic acid should reduce the amount of blood loss in obstetric surgeries [11]. Whereas this should be true among women with PAS as well, administration of tranexamic acid may indicate significant or ongoing blood loss, which triggers its administration, rather than being a risk factor for massive bleeding.

In fact, these concerns are common with machine learning models, which commonly use retrospective studies to provide sufficiently large databases for machine learning algorithms. Interestingly, data scientists do not necessarily consider that as a limitation. Unlike conventional statistics, machine learning does not investigate or highlight inference between a variable and an outcome. Instead, it builds models that use all complex interactions between all variables, including unrecognized ones, to predict an outcome. Thus, it does not necessarily define understandable or recognizable direct associations and should not be used for this propose. Indeed, they are meant to analyze the whole clinical scenario including all linked patient variables [12].

Finally, institutional auditing of these scores may be necessary since estimation of blood loss and admission to ICU may be influenced by institutional methods and protocols, respectively, and score interpretation may be adjusted based on internal outcomes.

Conservative Management of PAS (CON-PAS) Score

Score Development

CON-PAS score is a new scoring system that was designed to predict probability of success of uterus-preserving procedures in women with PAS prior to delivery [13]. The score was generated using the subset of women who underwent uterine preservation from the Placenta Accreta Spectrum International Database (PAS-ID), which was originally created to produce PAR scores [14]. Data from 587 women was included to develop this score using logistic regression approach [13].

Score Components

Composition of this score is similar to PAR-P score, where both antenatal and intraoperative factors are considered. Consequently, it predicts success of uterus-preserving procedures as per anticipated clinical scenarios at the time of surgery. The most contributing factors to this score are possibility of local uterine resection, number of previous cesarean deliveries, and type of uterine incision. In general, feasibility of local uterine resection and uterine incision away from placenta site contributes the most to uterine preservation success, while increasing number of previous cesarean deliveries and classic uterine incision are associated with increased risk of failed uterine preservation (Fig. 10.4).

Score Performance

According to the original study, AUC of this model in predicting success of uterine preservation was 0.91. The score was internally validated using a subset of data that was not involved in score creation (validation cohort) and AUC for this cohort was 0.90 [13]. Unpublished results on external validity of CON-PAS score, based on the

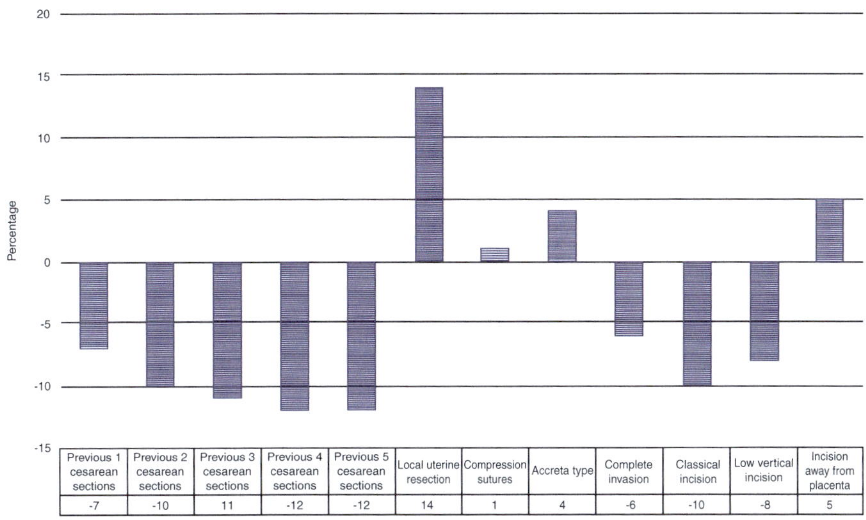

Fig. 10.4 Factors included in CON-PAS score and their magnitude of contribution

same database used to validate PAR-A score, showed that AUC of this prospective cohort was 0.94.

Score Applicability

The score was built using traditional logistic regression models. However, a software is available to determine probability of procedure success and plot the score in comparison to reference score ranges in women who had successful versus unsuccessful uterine preservation procedures (MoggeSoft®); (MoggeSoft For medical software, Egypt) [15].

Although the score seems to be a unique tool to counsel women and determine whether they are good candidates for uterine preservation, some of the information used to calculate CON-PAS is only determined intraoperatively. Accordingly, it may be used to determine potential probability of success if certain criteria are met or not met during surgery. Thereby, a decision may be altered based on intraoperative assessment in correspondence to previously calculated scores. For example, the score may indicate high probability of treatment success if local uterine resection or incision away from placental site can be achieved. Otherwise, hysterectomy should be better performed. Obviously, using the score in such a way may be complex, yet beneficial in certain scenarios. Also, some intraoperative findings may be anticipated through prenatal and intraoperative imaging.

Disadvantages and Limitations

Similar to PAR score, the score emerged from a retrospective study. Nevertheless, the score is more transparent and simple compared to machine learning-based scores. Therefore, association between variables and score outcome is interpretable. As mentioned earlier, practical applicability of CON-PAS score may not be straightforward since it consider alternative plans based on intraoperative findings. In addition, PAS-ID, the original database, originated from centers that possess long experience in uterine preservation, and results should not be generalized to less experienced centers, even if calculated scores are reassuring.

Conclusion

Recently, novel scores have been proposed to predict perioperative outcomes in women with PAS. Specifically, PAR scores are designed to calculate risk of adverse outcomes at time of cesarean delivery, while CON-PAS score predicts the chance of uterine preservation success. These types of scores have not previously available and their potential implementation is new to the field of PAS management. Wide application of these scores may enhance their validity as a tool that aids patient counseling, decision-making, and management planning.

References

1. Poder L, Weinstein S, Maturen KE, Feldstein VA, Mackenzie DC, Oliver ER, et al. ACR appropriateness criteria® placenta Accreta Spectrum disorder. J Am Coll Radiol: JACR. 2020;17(5s):S207–s14.
2. Jauniaux E, Chantraine F, Silver RM, Langhoff-Roos J. FIGO consensus guidelines on placenta accreta spectrum disorders: epidemiology. Int J Gynaecol Obstet. 2018;140(3):265–73.
3. Ali H, Chandraharan E. Etiopathogenesis and risk factors for placental accreta spectrum disorders. Best Pract Res Clin Obstet Gynaecol. 2021;72:4–12.
4. Jauniaux E, Kingdom JC, Silver RM. A comparison of recent guidelines in the diagnosis and management of placenta accreta spectrum disorders. Best Pract Res Clin Obstet Gynaecol. 2021;72:102–16.
5. Carusi DA. The placenta accreta spectrum: epidemiology and risk factors. Clin Obstet Gynecol. 2018;61(4):733–42.
6. Jauniaux E, Ayres-de-Campos D, Langhoff-Roos J, Fox KA, Collins S, Diagnosis FPA, et al. FIGO classification for the clinical diagnosis of placenta accreta spectrum disorders. Int J Gynecol Obstet. 2019;146(1):20–4.
7. Shazly SA, Hortu I, Shih J-C, Melekoglu R, Fan S, Ahmed FA, et al. Prediction of clinical outcomes in women with placenta accreta spectrum using machine learning models: an international multicenter study. J Matern Fetal Neonatal Med. 2021:1–10.
8. Shazly SA, Anan MA, Makukhina TB, Melekoglu R, Ahmed FA, Pinto PV, et al. Placenta accreta risk–antepartum score in predicting clinical outcomes of placenta accreta spectrum: a multicenter validation study. Int J Gynecol Obstet. 2021;158(2):424–31.

9. Cover T, Hart P. Nearest neighbor pattern classification. IEEE Trans Inf Theory. 1967;13(1):21–7.
10. Trevethan R. Sensitivity, specificity, and predictive values: foundations, pliabilities, and pitfalls in research and practice. Front Public Health. 2017;5:307.
11. Sentilhes L, Sénat MV, Le Lous M, Winer N, Rozenberg P, Kayem G, et al. Tranexamic acid for the prevention of blood loss after cesarean delivery. N Engl J Med. 2021;384(17):1623–34.
12. Rajula HSR, Verlato G, Manchia M, Antonucci N, Fanos VJM. Comparison of conventional statistical methods with machine learning in medicine: diagnosis, drug development, and treatment. Medicina (Kaunas). 2020;56(9):455.
13. Shazly SA, Hortu I, Shih JC, Melekoglu R, Fan S, Ahmed FA, et al. Prediction of success of uterus-preserving management in women with placenta accreta spectrum (CON-PAS score): a multicenter international study. Int J Gynecol Obstet. 2021;154(2):304–11.
14. Goldenberg SL, Nir G, Salcudean SE. A new era: artificial intelligence and machine learning in prostate cancer. Nat Rev Urol. 2019;16(7):391–403.
15. Kotsiantis SB, Zaharakis I, Pintelas P. Supervised machine learning: a review of classification techniques. Emerging artificial intelligence applications in computer engineering. Informatica. 2007;160(1):3–24.

Chapter 11
Evidence-Based Management of Placenta Accreta Spectrum

Sherif A. Shazly, Ahmad A. Radwan, AlBatool M. AlMahdy, Mohamed I. Ateya, Mostafa H. Abouzeid, Esraa G. Sayed, and Gena M. Elassall

Introduction

Since PAS was first prescribed in the first half of the twentieth century, hysterectomy has been the sole management of this life-threatening disorder for several decades [1]. Uterus-preserving procedures have not been endorsed until relatively recently, perhaps in concordance with our developing understanding of risk factors and antenatal diagnosis, which has rendered planned delivery feasible for many cases. However, uterus-preserving procedures comprise a spectrum of expanding inconsistent techniques that are associated with variable success rates and complications [2–4]. These procedures are highly dependent on surgeon's experience and dexterity, and evidence on their safety and efficacy is limited. In addition, some of these procedures may include manual removal of the placenta, which makes such procedures concerning since this may trigger extensive and life-threatening bleeding. Although uterus-preserving procedures have been increasingly appraised as a possible alternative particularly in women who are highly motivated to maintain their fertility, caesarean hysterectomy remains the standard procedure and is universally recommended by internationally recognized practice guidelines especially in severe cases [5].

S. A. Shazly (✉)
Department of Obstetrics and Gynecology, Leeds Teaching Hospitals NHS Trust, Leeds, UK
e-mail: sherif.shazly@nhs.net

A. A. Radwan · A. M. AlMahdy · E. G. Sayed · G. M. Elassall
Faculty of Medicine, Assiut University, Assiut, Egypt

M. I. Ateya
Department of Obstetrics and Gynecology, South Valley University, Qena, Egypt

M. H. Abouzeid
Department of Obstetrics and Gynecology, Assiut University, Assiut, Egypt

S. A. Shazly, A. A. Nassr (eds.), *Placenta Accreta Spectrum*,
https://doi.org/10.1007/978-3-031-10347-6_11

Although evidence-based recommendations on management of PAS disorders have been consistently adopted by several international communities, this topic lacks high-quality prospective studies that would support many of these recommendations [4]. This may be due to the low incidence of PAS (0.2% of all pregnancies), which precludes conduction of large studies [6]. Furthermore, the serious nature of PAS disorders creates ethical restrictions to clinical assessment of some management approaches. In addition, many studies reflect a particular team-based practice on selected group of cases (case series) rather than a comprehensive and universal protocol to all women with PAS. Therefore, reproducibility of emerging results is usually doubtful. Unfortunately, external validation of any of the proposed techniques, on a larger cohort or in a different setting, is rarely done. These concerns disrupt robustness of evidence and broaden the gap between evidence-based guidance and actual practice since none of the these practice-based approaches could be satisfactorily studied to prove its safety and efficacy.

Evidence-Based Recommendations on Management of PAS

Antenatal Screening

With the rising trend of cesarean section rates worldwide, PAS is no longer considered a rare disorder. The Royal College of Obstetricians and Gynaecologists (RCOG) highlights the importance of identifying PAS risk factors during antenatal assessment [7]. Antenatal suspicion of PAS facilitates planned management, which yields substantially better outcomes compared to unrecognized cases diagnosed at the time of labor. Therefore, the Society of Obstetricians and Gynaecologists of Canada (SOGC) recommends routine screening of women with prior cesarean delivery or uterine surgery for PAS [8]. Screening can be made using ultrasound, which is ideally performed at the time of mid-trimester fetal anatomy scan [8]. As recommended by the Royal Australian and New Zealand College of Obstetricians and Gynaecologists (RANZCOG), suspected cases of PAS should be planned as confirmed PAS and should be referred to a PAS specialized center [9].

Transfer of Care

Standard management of women with PAS should be initiated as early as suspicion is raised. The American College of Obstetricians and Gynecologists (ACOG) recommends immediate transfer of suspected patients to a tertiary center that has the facility to follow up and manage women with PAS disorders [6, 10]. Specifically, PAS referral centers should have sufficient and readily available blood products. Availability of autologous blood salvage devices is preferred. Autologous cell salvage is associated with lower need for allogenic blood transfusion, with no increased risk of complications [11–13]. Therefore, the International Federation of Gynecology and Obstetrics (FIGO) recommends the use of autologous cell salvage when available [14]. Indeed, autologous cell salvage may be compulsory if women decline or cannot receive blood products, e.g., Jehovah's Witnesses [15, 16].

Furthermore, PAS specialized centers should support PAS-directed multidisciplinary care, which consists of an obstetrician or obstetric surgeon, a pelvic surgeon, an anesthesiologist, an intensivist, a neonatologist, a urologist, a hematologist, and an interventional radiologist [17]. Multidisciplinary structure, involved in decision-making and clinical care, promotes cumulative institutional experience in all aspects of PAS management, which eventually results in significant improvement of maternal outcomes and quality of care [18]. Specifically, this mounting experience yields lower risk of massive blood transfusion, intensive care admission, and reoperation [19]. Similar recommendations are made by the SOGC, which supports the role of specialized centers and multidisciplinary approach to optimize care of women with PAS [8]. SOGC defines the structure of these centers and emphasizes on the necessity of level II obstetric ultrasonography, level III maternity unit, level II neonatal intensive care unit, and adult intensive care unit. The role of centers of excellence and multidisciplinary care in reducing maternal morbidity is also recognized by FIGO [14, 17, 20–22]. In addition, FIGO strongly recommends that a surgeon specialized in complex pelvic surgery attends delivery [14]. A retrospective study of 98 women showed that attendance of a gynecologic oncologist was associated with less blood loss and lower need for blood transfusion [23]. Similarly, RCOG endorses the role of complex pelvic surgeons as a part of the managing team [7].

The managing team should hold a thorough discussion with the patient to explain her potential diagnosis. Women should be counseled on different management scenarios and potential complications associated with PAS including massive bleeding and potential need for blood transfusion, urinary tract injury, and hysterectomy and additional procedures that may be necessary to manage these complications. RCOG also recommends that anesthesia plan should be discussed antenatally and women should be counseled and consented on the possibility of conversion from spinal to general anesthesia [7].

Delivery Planning

Planned delivery is a crucial part of PAS management and is associated with better outcomes compared to emergency delivery [24, 25]. Delivery should be scheduled on a date that weighs the risk of preterm labor against risk of emergency delivery. According to ACOG, patient preference and maternal and fetal status should be also considered. Accordingly, "34 weeks" may be the optimal time to schedule delivery unless earlier delivery is otherwise indicated [26, 27]. Delivery window may be extended to 36 + 0 weeks. However, ACOG does not support expectant management beyond this point because it may increase risk of spontaneous bleeding and emergency delivery [26]. For similar reasons, SOGC recommends elective delivery between 34 and 36 weeks of gestation. Antenatal steroids should be offered within 1 week of planned delivery if it is scheduled at or before 34^{+6} weeks of gestation [8, 28]. FIGO also considers the balance between risks of bleeding and prematurity and recommends scheduled delivery, preferably between 34 and 35 weeks [20, 29–31]. However, RCOG extends the window of scheduled delivery between 35^{+0} and 36^{+6} weeks of gestation [7]. This recommendation is supported by retrospective data which did not show significant risks associated with expectant management of PAS beyond 36 weeks [32]. An emergency plan should be readily available if immediate delivery is necessary for bleeding or other urgent obstetric indications. SOGC recommends that women are counseled not to travel far away from specialized centers. They should be provided with a document declaring their diagnosis, managing center, and plan of care to facilitate their transfer in case of emergency [8].

As a part of planned delivery, operative room should be equipped with available blood products, and the blood bank should be notified and should anticipate and prepare for massive transfusion protocols. Devices and medications required for management of postpartum hemorrhage should be readily accessible. Management approach should be thoroughly discussed with the patient in advance, and she should be counseled on the necessity, complications, and outcomes of peripartum hysterectomy [10]. Women who are highly motivated to reserve future fertility should be aware of uterus-preserving options. ACOG recommends that decision should be individualized [10]. However, counseling should be prudently made since these options are not supported by high-quality evidence and they may be associated with significant risks. Either way, women should be consented for hysterectomy since uterus-preserving procedures are liable to failure or infeasibility due to intraoperative bleeding. It is important to emphasize that there are no randomized clinical trials or prospective well-controlled observational studies that compare planned hysterectomy to uterus-preserving procedures and current data is mostly derived from single-arm and small studies [33].

Although planned delivery in a specialized tertiary center is indicated in all suspected cases, unexpected intraoperative diagnosis of PAS is common, reaching more than 30% of all cases in some reports originating from developed countries [34]. In these situations, ACOG recommends proceeding with uterine closure and hysterectomy. Unfortunately, hysterectomy may not be feasible in all birth units, and under these circumstances, women should be hemodynamically stabilized with blood transfusion, tranexamic acid infusion, and abdominal packing if necessary, before the patient is transferred to a specialized center [10]. Similarly, if PAS is recognized prior to uterine incision, SOGC recommends that the abdomen should be closed, and the patient should be immediately transferred to a specialized center for definitive management [8, 35].

Unexpected intraoperative diagnosis of PAS may occur after vaginal delivery even in the absence of risk factors. If the placenta is retained with no uterine bleeding indicating placental separation, and no plane of placental separation can be felt by bimanual examination, PAS disorder should be suspected. According to SOGC guidelines, the acceptable approach comprises cutting of the umbilical cord and clamping it with an absorbable suture, administration of intravenous prophylactic antibiotics, and keeping an intravenous access with continuous oxytocin infusion. Oral intake is prevented for 12–24 hours should general anesthesia be needed for urgent surgical management. According to SOGC, placental tissue may be removed under ultrasound or hysteroscopic guidance if the patient remains stable with no active bleeding [8]. High-intensity focused ultrasound has been recently proposed in stable women if retained placental tissue is larger than 3 cm, yet not occupying more than half of the uterine cavity [36].

Preoperative Preparation

As a part of planned management, optimization of perioperative environment should be contemplated. Antenatal suspicion of PAS provides sufficient time to review medical records, request additional information, and carry out any necessary measures. SOGC recommends maternal serology testing, including hepatitis C, hepatitis B, and HIV viruses prior to delivery. Additionally, previous surgical reports, especially if associated with massive blood transfusion, should be obtained. A simple but crucial measurement is correction and follow-up of maternal hemoglobin prior to delivery since anemia may aggravate sequalae of blood loss both quantitatively and qualitatively [8]. Iron deficiency is the most common cause of anemia in pregnancy and can be corrected either orally or intravenously [37]. FIGO also proposes the use of erythropoietin, if clinically indicated, understanding that this treatment is associated with significantly higher cost [14].

Since PAS-indicated cesarean hysterectomy is associated with high incidence of urinary tract injuries (approximately one third of cases), utility of preoperative placement of ureteric stents has been investigated and was found to reduce the incidence of urinary tract injury to 6% [38]. Therefore, ureteric stents are endorsed by FIGO and RANZCOG particularly if bladder invasion is preoperatively suspected [9, 14]. Similarly, RCOG does not support the use of ureteric stents and cystoscopy unless the bladder is likely invaded [7, 39, 40]. Preoperative cystoscopy may be considered to assess bladder invasion [39]. A full bladder may facilitate bladder dissection from the lower segment, cystotomy, and cervical identification when total hysterectomy is performed [31]. Therefore, RCOG recommends bladder filling to identify bladder separation plane and cystotomy to excise affected area when bladder invasion is confirmed [7, 40, 41].

Massive bleeding and blood transfusion are the most common complications of PAS, and cross-matched blood products should be readily available for planned and emergency delivery. Obstetric hemorrhage in PAS patients requires greater compensation for the lost blood compared to other causes of postpartum hemorrhage. Therefore, RCOG recommends that standardized PAS-directed national or institutional protocols of postpartum hemorrhage and blood transfusion should be adopted and strictly followed [7, 42–44].

Intraoperative Management

I. *Anesthesia*

As recommended by FIGO, the type of anesthesia should be determined by the anesthetist in collaboration with the multidisciplinary team especially when risk of massive intraoperative bleeding is significant [14]. However, if diagnosis of PAS is made intraoperatively, the probability of conversion of regional to general anesthesia is high [45–48]. General anesthesia is more suitable in emergency situations where anesthesia can be established quickly, and resuscitation of unstable women is facilitated. In general, regional anesthesia is preferable to general anesthesia whenever feasible since it is associated with lower incidence of anesthetic complications. Although some studies showed that regional anesthesia may reduce maternal morbidity caused by hemorrhage and blood transfusion in women with PAS [49, 50], a retrospective study of 50 cases with PAS did not support this conclusion [48]. In addition, regional anesthesia precludes the risk of neonatal respiratory depression caused by volatile drugs that cross the placenta. Fortunately, this risk may not be substantially significant [48].

II. *Positioning*

Intraoperative placement of women with PAS in a modified lithotomy position is preferred. SOGC endorses this position should vaginal access be needed and to facilitate monitoring of vaginal bleeding intraoperatively [8].

III. *Perioperative Medications*

Antibiotics and tranexamic acid should be administered intravenously at the time of skin incision [8, 51]. Oral or intravenous administration of tranexamic acid pre- or intraoperatively is also highly recommended by FIGO based on established results of a large double-blinded clinical trial. The study, that comprised 20,060 women, showed that use of tranexamic acid reduces postpartum hemorrhage-related deaths with no increased risks of thromboembolism [52]. Although the study was not specific to PAS, women with placenta previa or accreta were not excluded from the study, and they presented 9% of the study population.

IV. *Skin Incision*

Classically, the pelvis should be accessed through a midline vertical skin incision. According to FIGO, midline skin incision should be opted for placentas that extend beyond the lower uterine segment toward the umbilicus and when cesarean hysterectomy is planned. However, transverse skin incision, either low or midline, may be appropriate depending on the highest level of anterior placental edge [53].

V. *Bladder Dissection*

Since urinary tract injuries can significantly complicate surgery and disrupt visualization of the field, FIGO recommends assessment of bladder invasion and proper bladder dissection before the fetus is delivered [38, 54]. This should be completed and diagnosis of percreta is confirmed before cystotomy and excision of the invaded area of bladder are made [53]. In such cases, a posterior approach may be required to facilitate uterine devascularization and hysterectomy [55].

VI. *Uterine Incision*
While assessing for extent of invasion, the uterus should be gently handled. Ultrasound can be used intraoperatively to guide uterine incision, which should be ideally a classical incision and should avoid cutting through the placenta. Intraoperative ultrasound has gained increasing popularity in localizing the placenta before uterine incision is made and is endorsed by SOGC and FIGO [8, 53]. Uterine incisions should be made above the upper placental margin including fundal hysterotomy which may be performed transversally to deliver the fetus if the placenta extends anteriorly [20, 21, 41, 56, 57]. Although the use of uterine staplers or Smith-Opitz clamps, as adopted in fetal surgery, may reduce intraoperative bleeding, availability and cost of these instruments limit the popularity of their application. SOGC recommends a one-layer closure of the uterus before proceeding with hysterectomy to reduce intraoperative blood loss [8].

VII. *Uterine Preservation*
Although ACOG endorses cesarean hysterectomy as the standard management of women with PAS, uterine preservation may be considered on individual basis [6, 10]. ACOG restricts uterine preservation to PAS associated with focal invasion where the adherent area is sufficiently localized to permit manual or surgical removal of the placenta with closure of the defect [27]. Similarly, RCOG considers partial myometrial resection if minimal invasion is identified. However, a consent to preserve the uterus should be obtained [7]. En bloc removal of placental invasion, followed by uterine repair, may be considered with larger adherent areas [58]. Accordingly, feasibility of uterine preservation is mainly determined intraoperatively. Therefore, women should be clearly counseled that even if uterine preservation would be considered, hysterectomy may be eventually warranted.

Extirpative technique of uterine preservation refers to manual or forceful removal of the placenta to empty the uterus followed by bleeding control. Although the technique is old and well known in management of postpartum bleeding associated with incomplete separation of the placenta [15, 59–64], it is associated with substantial risk of intractable uterine bleeding in the presence of PAS, which would double the average blood loss in these cases [64]. Compared to "leaving placenta in situ," extirpative technique is associated with higher incidence of blood transfusion, disseminated intravascular coagulopathy (DIC), hysterectomy, and infections [65]. Therefore, FIGO recommends avoidance of extirpative technique and advises against manual removal of the placenta if PAS is suspected and/or placental separation does not easily occur [53].

In concordance with ACOG, SOGC also considers uterine preservation if the placenta is separable with focal invasion that can be excised and repaired. In fact, excision of invaded myometrium may also reduce risk of recurrence in subsequent pregnancies [66]. Although FIGO realizes focal resection and reconstruction of the uterus as a possible method of uterine preservation [53, 58, 67, 68], it raises a valid concern on its reproducibility since the procedure could be highly dependent on surgeon's skills [53]. SOGC also endorses a technique of perioperative localization of placenta wedge which may be guided by preoperative magnetic resonance imaging (MRI), pelvic devascularization, and placental nonseparation with resection of the invaded wedge. This procedure is known as "triple-P technique" [8, 69]. Although triple-P technique seems to reduce the incidence of hysterectomy, data may be too sparse to make a strong recommendation [69, 70]. FIGO also endorses the promising results of placental bed tamponade, which involves suturing of the inverted cervical lips to the lower uterine wall. The procedure was efficient as indicated by a few case series [71–76]. Nevertheless, larger studies may be warranted to establish robust recommendations. Both triple-P procedure and cervical tamponade were not considered by the RCOG due to limited evidence [7]. Uterine compression sutures have been proposed as a procedure to preserve the uterus in certain situations. They include either the same compression sutures used to manage atonic postpartum hemorrhage (e.g., B-Lynch sutures) or other sutures designed specifically to control bleeding from placental bed (e.g., multiple 8 compression sutures) [71, 77]. Although these procedures may be associated with reported cases of wound infection and intrauterine synechiae, overall, they seem safe and associated with reassuring long-term fertility outcomes [78–80]. However, most data originate from case series and small studies, and evidence is too limited to recommend their implementation [81]. A retrospective study of 148 women showed that the use of Bakri balloon for uterine preservation was comparable to local uterine wall resection and hysterectomy in rate of admission to intensive care unit, duration of hospital stay, operative time, and amount of transfused blood products [82]. However, larger well-designed studies are warranted to validate these conclusions. In fact, data on many uterus-preserving procedures are derived from case series and small studies and may be associated with inconsistent outcomes [83].

SOGC also acknowledges an alternative to hysterectomy if non-focal invasion is found. In this situation, there should be no trial to remove the placenta, which is left in place and the uterus is closed. Leaving "placenta in situ" is the first established uterus-preserving procedure. In this method, the cord is cut away from its placental origin and the uterus is closed [53]. Thereafter, patients expectantly managed awaiting tissue atrophy secondary to reduction in blood supply with subsequent resorption, separation, and expulsion of placental segments [84]. In a French retrospective multicenter study of 167 patients managed with this approach, success rate was 78% and the uterus took a median of 13.5 weeks (range 4–60) to spontaneously empty [85]. Although this approach is recognized by SOGC and RANZCOG, they are obvious about its drawbacks, which should be clearly shared with the patient before a preoperative decision is made. They include prolonged recovery course, relatively long follow-up, and persistent possibility of secondary hysterectomy (up to 40%), which may be indicated up to several months after delivery [3, 8, 9, 83]. Furthermore, leaving placenta in situ can lead to significant maternal morbidities. Pelvic infection, sepsis, hemorrhage, coagulopathy, and pulmonary embolism are among the reported complications of this approach [2, 15, 85, 86]. FIGO and RCOG state that administration of prophylactic antibiotics may be considered if the placenta is left in situ. Nevertheless, level of evidence is low [7, 27, 53]. Administration of methotrexate, as an adjuvant treatment to accelerate placental autolysis, was not shown to be considerably effective based on data from small studies and was associated with significant side effects such as pancytopenia and nephrotoxicity. In addition, methotrexate may increase risk of pelvic infection and sepsis due to its immunosuppressive effect [87–91]. Therefore, FIGO and RCOG recommend against the use of methotrexate if the placenta is left in situ [7, 53]. Postpartum removal of placental tissue using hysteroscopy and ultrasound guidance has been proposed to hasten placental resolution [92, 93]. However, these options are only supported by limited data, and risk of perforation of a postpartum uterus presents a major concern to their use [92]. High-intensity focused ultrasound, as a method to ablate placental tissue without perforation risk, has been recently proposed with initial promising results [94]. However, this method has only been investigated in women with residual placental tissue larger than 3 cm, but not occupying greater than 50% of the uterine cavity and has not been investigated in women who were managed specifically by leaving the whole placenta in situ [36].

VIII. *Cesarean Hysterectomy*

If cesarean hysterectomy is planned, placental removal should not be attempted. Leaving the placenta in place while proceeding with hysterectomy is associated with less blood loss and lower incidence of blood transfusion [29, 32, 95, 96]. Although this practice is recommended by FIGO and RCOG, FIGO also considers a gentle trial to remove the placenta acceptable if spontaneous separation occurs or if placental invasion appears minimal [41]. In absence of spontaneous separation, FIGO advises that uterotonics should not be administered and that the operative team should proceed with immediate hysterectomy [14]. FIGO also recommends total hysterectomy over subtotal hysterectomy. Although subtotal hysterectomy is associated with shorter operative time, less blood loss and lower rate of blood transfusion, cervical involvement by placental invasion and risk of cancers that may rise from cervical stump make subtotal hysterectomy less preferred in modern practice [14]. Nevertheless, the Society of Maternal-Fetal Medicine (SMFM) survey showed balanced predilection among surgeons regarding their preferred hysterectomy technique (55% for total hysterectomy vs. 45% for subtotal hysterectomy) [97]. Other modifications to hysterectomy including posterior retrograde hysterectomy via pouch of Douglas [98], modified radical hysterectomy with the use of bipolar cautery device [20], linear cutting stable device for hysterotomy [99], and use of vessel-sealing devices [100] were also described.

In some cases, the placenta may extensively invade the surrounding pelvic organs, and thereby, immediate hysterectomy may become challenging to perform. Delayed hysterectomy may be scheduled from the 3rd to the 12th week after delivery [21, 101, 102]. The rationale of delayed surgery is to allow tissue resorption and reduction of vascularity before hysterectomy is performed. FIGO endorses the option of delayed hysterectomy if immediate hysterectomy is not feasible understanding that level of evidence, supporting this practice, is low [14]. Total blood loss associated with delayed surgery may be comparable to immediate hysterectomy [21, 101, 103]. However, delayed hysterectomy may be associated with risks of leaving placenta in situ. Thus, regular follow-up is mandatory and emergency hysterectomy should be planned, if necessary [14].

IX. *Pelvic Devascularization*

In conjugation with primary intervention, pelvic devascularization is considered by many surgeons to reduce blood loss. Although internal iliac artery ligation is adopted by many PAS specialized centers, the procedure has not been proved to be effective [8]. This is probably because the rich collateral blood supply from external iliac arteries and the aorta compensates for internal iliac artery occlusion. Furthermore, internal iliac artery ligation may add to complexity of surgery and may be associated with longer operative time and risk of vascular complications [104]. Preoperative bilateral transfemoral placement of internal iliac artery balloons, which are inflated intraoperatively after delivering the fetus, was associated with similar outcomes [105, 106]. Thus, both techniques of occlusion are not routinely recommended by the SOGC [8]. Similarly, FIGO does not recommend routine radiologic or surgical devascularization [53]. In addition to their limited effectiveness, these procedures are associated with several complications including popliteal and external iliac arteries thrombosis [107, 108], rupture of iliac artery [109], and nerve injury due to ischemia.

Emerging evidence on temporary infrarenal aortic balloon occlusion supports its safety and efficacy. A meta-analysis of 11 clinical studies (776 patients) showed that the procedure was associated with significant reduction in blood loss (mean difference [MD], 1480 ml; 95% confidence interval [CI], −1806 to −1154 ml), operative time (MD, 29.23 min; 95% CI, −46.04 to −12.42), and volume of blood transfusion (MD, 1125 ml; 95% CI −1264 to −987). The procedure was also associated with shorter hospitalization and lowered hysterectomy rate when performed alone with uterus-preserving procedures (OR 0.30, 95% CI 0.19 to 0.48) [110]. Therefore, this approach is recommended by SOGC particularly when a difficult surgery is anticipated [8]. Similarly, SMFM endorses clamping and balloon occlusion of abdominal aorta as an effective method to decrease pelvic blood flow. However, risk of potential distal thrombosis or ischemia should be considered, and a vascular surgeon should be consulted if this option is considered [111, 112]. RCOG highlights the controversial role of interventional radiology, including internal iliac artery, uterine artery, and aortic occlusion due to lack of large well-designed studies [113–122]. Nevertheless, RCOG considers this option in women who decline blood transfusion along with cell salvage [7, 43]. Arterial embolization may be considered in women with postpartum hemorrhage particularly if they are hemodynamically stable and do not suffer severe bleeding [123].

Postoperative Care

Postoperative care of women with PAS is crucial since complications of high-volume blood loss, prolonged surgery, intraoperative hypotension, and organ system dysfunctions are not uncommon. SMFM recommends frequent monitoring of vital signs and urine output using an indwelling catheter. If there is anuria or persistent hematuria, urinary tract injuries should be considered among other causes. Bleeding from the vagina and the incision should be frequently assessed. Anemias and coagulopathies should be corrected. Women should be encouraged to ambulate early to reduce risk of thromboembolic events associated with pregnancy, surgery, massive blood loss, and blood transfusion [111].

In women who were managed by "leaving placenta in situ," strict follow-up is indicated since residual villi may take up to 6 months to resolve [89]. There are no standardized protocols to follow up these patients. Nevertheless, follow-up should take place in a specialized center with suitable experience [53]. FIGO recommends weekly measurement of serum β-hCG to ensure reduction of placental tissue. Nevertheless, ultrasound remains the primary method of assessment of placental mass. Other imaging modalities, such as magnetic resonance imaging, are not required [124]. Besides, follow-up visits should include clinical assessment of vaginal bleeding and infection and investigations, such as vaginal culture, hemoglobin level, and leucocytic count, if indicated [85]. If postpartum course remains uncomplicated after 3 months, follow-up visits can be scheduled monthly [53].

Barriers to Evidence-Based Practice: Why Does Global Practice Not Strictly Follow Guidelines?

According to the World Health Organization (WHO), guidelines are a set of evidence-based recommendations that instruct clinicians on how to practice in a way that yields the best possible outcomes according to the highest quality of research [125, 126]. Although practice guidelines have played a major role in modern medicine, there are some inherent concerns that limit their reflection on clinical practice. For example, guidelines are associated with high dependency on homogenous controlled studies which may not be reflective of general population and actual practice circumstances. Also, guidelines tend to refer to committees' opinion to resolve many inconclusive issues, which may be influenced by personal perspectives, institutional style of practice, served population, and availability of resources. Guidelines may limit the role of personal experience and appreciate study quality at the expense of unstudied population, which may differ significantly from the study cohort [127, 128]. Thus, these recommendations may offer a treatment of a specific disease rather than a particular patient [129–131]. In fact, the process of generation of practice guidelines may be influenced by the origin of the study, and in some situations, national guidelines may prioritize regional studies over international studies even if the later exhibit higher quality or larger cohorts [132]. Guidelines are limited by lack of high-quality data, which results in exclusion of several approaches, some of which may be efficient or deemed efficient based on unpublished institutional experience. Nevertheless, evidence-based guidelines remain the most widely acceptable method to practice standardized medicine in a controlled fashion. Otherwise, practice would be inconsistent, significantly impacted by providers' varying experience, and medical malpractice will be challenging to define [29, 133].

Implementation of PAS guidelines may be challenged by several regional and clinical obstacles. Specifically, planned cesarean hysterectomy is defined as the standard management of PAS by all internationally recognizable practice guidelines. This is primarily due to safety concerns, which place a well-established surgery superior to less known and surgeon-dependent procedures. However, hysterectomy may have significant psychological sequalae in many women, including depression, even in the absence of preexisting psychiatric illness [134–136]. It is not uncommon that women experience negative thoughts regarding their physical and sexual well-being [137]. These sequalae are usually a reaction to their frustration of losing a special feminine organ and their inability to carry a pregnancy in the future. In some regions, the situation may be much exaggerated by cultural beliefs, lack of understanding and support, and restrictions to fertility options, particularly surrogacy. Under these circumstances, hysterectomy is strongly declined by many patients. Surgeons have had to establish their own experience in preserving the uterus to meet their patients' interests, and with time, uterus-preserving procedures have become more prevalent than hysterectomy in these regions. Therefore, some institutes may be concerned that practice guidelines preclude their expertise and enforce recommendations that present others' experiences. The varying intraoperative findings, endorsed by surgeons' experience, may not be recognized as efficiently by guidelines, which are limited by available studies, which do not necessarily present all clinical data [44, 86].

On the contrary, some evidence-based recommendations are derived from studies, conducted in highly equipped institutes, and recruited highly compliant women. Although these studies may provide evidence of high quality, their results may be challenging to reproduce or concerning to adopt. For example, "leaving the placenta in situ" is an acceptable approach for uterine preservation by many international guidelines and is supported over many other approaches that are globally more prevalent, yet less studied. Nevertheless, "leaving the placenta in situ" is seldom performed as indicated by surveys that screen experts' preference in management of PAS [97, 138, 139]. This may be attributed, in part, to complexity of follow-up and prolonged recovery course associated with this approach. In addition, many providers may be inconvenient with risks of serious complications, especially if patient compliance or institutional experience cannot be granted.

A survey of 36 experts in 2017, mainly based in Europe and Asia, showed that 61% perform primary cesarean hysterectomy as their first-line approach compared to 39% who opt for uterus-preserving procedures as a routine practice. Twenty eight percent of experts use partial myometrial resection and 17% use cervical tamponade. Atrial embolization is used by 50% of experts and 47% use intra-arterial balloons. In addition, 17 % of participants use methotrexate in their protocols [138]. This practice does not show substantial consistency with internationally recognized guidelines. Indeed, PAS practice is globally inconsistent, and data derived from different regions may vary. In a survey involving 508 of SMFM members, 14.9% report performing uterus-preserving procedures [139]. Nevertheless, data from the same region may not be consistent as well [97].

Validity of Established Practice: Why Does Established Practice Not Steer Guidelines?

As previously discussed, cesarean hysterectomy is considered the treatment of choice and the safest surgical approach in cases of PAS. However, international surveys revealed that many obstetricians consider uterus-preserving approaches their primary management of PAS even if not supported by evidence-based recommendations [138, 139]. Despite numerous studies that appraise a variety of uterus preserving procedures, none of these procedures has been recognized as a standard management by current guidelines [140–142]. This fact highlights the gap between evidence-based guidelines and actual practice in many regions although clinical studies, used to create evidence, are anticipated to emerge from and appraise contemporary practice.

One of the main explanations of this gap is rarity of the condition, which makes it challenging for obstetricians to investigate their proposed approaches on a large population. A recent review of conservative managements of PAS reported that 54% and 89% of available studies recruited less than 20 patients and less than 50 patients, respectively [36]. These small studies may only show descriptive results and may not be eligible for more robust statistical analysis, which is required to yield definite conclusions such as regression analysis. Similarly, experimental approaches are almost always tested through single-arm studies with small sample sizes or case series [143, 144]. To a large extent, PAS is inherently deprived of randomized clinical trials, which provide a high level of evidence, due to difficult recruitment and ethical restrictions to experimental research in life-threatening conditions. Prospective studies are not commonly conducted, probably due to difficult requirement as well. Thus, poor quality of most published data limits their impact on evidence-based guidelines [145–147].

Case reports and case series are frequently reported particularly to assess novel approaches in management of PAS [71, 146–153]. Again, these studies permit limited statistical inference. Moreover, they typically review a few surgeon-selected cases who were managed by a particular approach rather than a controlled study of all eligible women with definite preoperative and intraoperative selection criteria that permit reproducibility of outcomes. This type of studies is highly subjected to publication bias since authors may document cases that went well rather than those who had major complications or even died, resulting in possible underreporting of complications of these procedures. Many of the published procedures are surgeon- or institution-based, meaning that they convey their established experience, which may not be easily reproduced if a novice team tries the same approach. Moreover, studying these procedures by a different team in a different institute is unlikely to receive ethical approval given the limited supportive data of their safety.

For similar reasons, systematic reviews on PAS studies are limited. Trials to review available data to build stronger conclusions are confronted with significant heterogeneity in study design and outcomes [36, 140, 142, 154]. Many of these studies are associated with significant concerns such as considering missing information as a non-occurred event [140]. Several novel procedures are proposed and appraised with only a few of them undergoing further validation by other investigators, resulting in numerous isolated techniques associated with limited data. Assessment of long-term outcomes, including fertility outcomes, of most studies is deficient due to lack of long-term follow-up [141]. Documentation of degree of placental invasion and size of myometrial invasion is also deficient in many studies. Thereby, systematic reviews cannot confidently ascertain that a procedure can be safely recommended to all women with PAS [140, 142].

With scarcity of PAS patients, the amount of wasted data from unpublished cases remains a frustrating concern. A recent systematic review reported that all recent studies that investigated uterine preservation were conducted in 17 countries only, and more than 50% of them were conducted in China [36]. This indicates that current data are not presentative of global practice and that there is significant leak of precious information since most institutes do not publish their data. The lack of PAS-focused clinical researchers in these institutes is the likely explanation.

These concerns highlight the importance of multicenter studies, which can solve recruitment issues and cohort size, and reach centers that do not participate in PAS research even if clinical researchers are not readily available in these centers. Large retrospective data can yield an acceptable level of evidence to guide further multicenter prospective studies or clinical trials without evoking significant ethical concerns. It remains an ongoing challenge that current recommendations do not provide definite preoperative and intraoperative criteria to determine eligibility for each management option. Thus, it is also important to evaluate a complete management protocol, rather than a procedure, where each management is considered based on certain criteria, in order to establish a safe platform for management of women with PAS.

Conclusion

Cesarean hysterectomy is the primary management in women with PAS. Uterus-preserving procedures should only be considered on individual basis and women should be carefully counseled on their possible risks. With the rising incidence of PAS cases, clinical researchers should actively collaborate to utilize expanding data in order to establish contemporary management plans. Future studies should consider the role of selective protocols rather than individual procedures, and multi-center studies should be more frequently conducted to overcome inherent limitations to PAS-related research.

References

1. Irving F. A study of placenta accreta. Surg Gynecol Obstet. 1937;64:178–200.
2. Clausen C, Lönn L, Langhoff-Roos J. Management of placenta percreta: a review of published cases. Acta Obstet Gynecol Scand. 2014;93(2):138–43.
3. Amsalem H, Kingdom JC, Farine D, Allen L, Yinon Y, D'Souza DL, et al. Planned caesarean hysterectomy versus "conserving" caesarean section in patients with placenta accreta. J Obstet Gynaecol Can. 2011;33(10):1005–10.
4. Jauniaux E, Collins SL, Jurkovic D, Burton GJ. Accreta placentation: a systematic review of prenatal ultrasound imaging and grading of villous invasiveness. Am J Obstet Gynecol. 2016;215(6):712–21.
5. Jauniaux E, Chantraine F, Silver R, Langhoff-Roos J, FIGO Placenta Accreta Diagnosis and Management Expert Consensus Panel. FIGO consensus guidelines on placenta accreta spectrum disorders: epidemiology. Int J Gynaecol Obstet. 2018;140(3):265–73.
6. Accreta P. Committee Opinion No. 529. American College of Obstetricians and Gynecologists. Obstet Gynecol. 2012;120:207–11.
7. Jauniaux E, Alfirevic Z, Bhide A, Belfort M, Burton G, Collins S, et al. Placenta praevia and placenta accreta: diagnosis and management: green-top guideline No. 27a. BJOG. 2019;126(1):e1–e48.
8. Hobson SR, Kingdom JC, Murji A, Windrim RC, Carvalho JC, Singh SS, et al. No. 383-screening, diagnosis, and management of placenta accreta spectrum disorders. J Obstet Gynaecol Can. 2019;41(7):1035–49.
9. Royal Australian and New Zealand College of Obstetricians and Gynaecologists. placenta accreta. https://ranzcog.edu.au/statements-guidelines/obstetrics/placenta-accreta-(c-obs-20). Accessed on Jan 20th, 2021. 2015
10. Cahill AG, Beigi R, Heine RP, Silver RM, Wax JR. Placenta Accreta Spectrum. Am J Obstet Gynecol. 2018;219(6):B2–B16.
11. McDonnell N, Kennedy D, Long L, Gallagher-Swann M, Paech MJ. The development and implementation of an obstetric cell salvage service. Anaesth Intensive Care. 2010;38(3):492–9.
12. Elagamy A, Abdelaziz A, Ellaithy M. The use of cell salvage in women undergoing cesarean hysterectomy for abnormal placentation. Int J Obstet Anesth. 2013;22(4):289–93.
13. Lew E. Tagore SJSmj. Implementation of an obstetric cell salvage service in a tertiary women's hospital. 2015;56(8):445.
14. Allen L, Jauniaux E, Hobson S, Papillon-Smith J, Belfort MA, Diagnosis FPA, et al. FIGO consensus guidelines on placenta accreta spectrum disorders: Nonconservative surgical management. Int J Gynaecol Obstet. 2018;140(3):281–90.

15. Chiang Y-C, Shih J-C, Lee C-N. Septic shock after conservative management for placenta accreta. Taiwan J Obstet Gynecol. 2006;45(1):64–6.
16. ACOG Practice Bulletin No. 95: anemia in pregnancy. Obstet Gynecol. 2008;112(1):201–7.
17. Eller AG, Bennett MA, Sharshiner M, Masheter C, Soisson AP, Dodson M, et al. Maternal morbidity in cases of placenta accreta managed by a multidisciplinary care team compared with standard obstetric care. Obstet Gynecol. 2011;117(2 Pt 1):331–7.
18. Shamshirsaz AA, Fox KA, Erfani H, Clark SL, Salmanian B, Baker BW, et al. Multidisciplinary team learning in the management of the morbidly adherent placenta: outcome improvements over time. Am J Obstet Gynecol. 2017;216(6):612. e1–5.
19. Smulian JC, Pascual A-L, Hesham H, Qureshey E, Bijoy Thomas M, Depuy AM, et al. Invasive placental disease: the impact of a multi-disciplinary team approach to management. J Matern Fetal Neonatal Med. 2017;30(12):1423–7.
20. Shamshirsaz AA, Fox KA, Salmanian B, Diaz-Arrastia CR, Lee W, Baker BW, et al. Maternal morbidity in patients with morbidly adherent placenta treated with and without a standardized multidisciplinary approach. Am J Obstet Gynecol. 2015;212(2):218. e1–9.
21. Al-Khan A, Gupta V, Illsley NP, Mannion C, Koenig C, Bogomol A, et al. Maternal and fetal outcomes in placenta accreta after institution of team-managed care. Reprod Sci. 2014;21(6):761–71.
22. Smulian JC, Pascual A-L, Hesham H, Qureshey E, Bijoy Thomas M. Depuy AM, et al. Invasive placental disease: the impact of a multi-disciplinary team approach to management. 2017;30(12):1423–7.
23. Brennan DJ, Schulze B, Chetty N, Crandon A, Petersen SG, Gardener G, et al. Surgical management of abnormally invasive placenta: a retrospective cohort study demonstrating the benefits of a standardized operative approach. Acta Obstet Gynecol Scand. 2015;94(12):1380–6.
24. Chestnut DH, Dewan DM, Redick LF, Caton D, Spielman FJ. Anesthetic management for obstetric hysterectomy: a multi-institutional study. Anesthesiology. 1989;70(4):607–10.
25. Eller A, Porter T, Soisson P, Silver R. Optimal management strategies for placenta accreta. BJOG Int J Obstet Gynaecol. 2009;116(5):648–54.
26. Angstmann T, Gard G, Harrington T, Ward E, Thomson A, Giles W. Surgical management of placenta accreta: a cohort series and suggested approach. Am J Obstet Gynecol. 2010;202(1):38. e1–9.
27. Fox KA, Shamshirsaz AA, Carusi D, Secord AA, Lee P, Turan OM, et al. Conservative management of morbidly adherent placenta: expert review. Am J Obstet Gynecol. 2015;213(6):755–60.
28. Skoll A, Boutin A, Bujold E, Burrows J, Crane J, Geary M, et al. No. 364-antenatal corticosteroid therapy for improving neonatal outcomes. J Obstet Gynaecol Can. 2018;40(9):1219–39.
29. Eller A, Porter T, Soisson P, Silver RM. Optimal management strategies for placenta accreta. BJOG. 2009;116(5):648–54.
30. Warshak CR, Ramos GA, Eskander R, Benirschke K, Saenz CC, Kelly TF, et al. Effect of predelivery diagnosis in 99 consecutive cases of placenta accreta. Obstet Gynecol. 2010;115(1):65–9.
31. Seoud M, Nasr R, Berjawi G, Zaatari G, Seoud T, Shatila A, et al. Placenta accreta: Elective versus emergent delivery as a major predictor of blood loss. J Neonatal Perinatal Med. 2017;10(1):9–15.
32. Belfort MA. Indicated preterm birth for placenta accreta. Seminars in perinatology. Elsevier; 2011.
33. Jauniaux E, Hussein AM, Fox KA, Collins SL. New evidence-based diagnostic and management strategies for placenta accreta spectrum disorders. Best Pract Res Clin Obstet Gynaecol. 2019;61:75–88.
34. Rosenbloom JI, Hirshberg JS, Stout MJ, Cahill AG, Macones GA, Tuuli MG. Clinical Diagnosis of placenta Accreta and Clinicopathological outcomes. Am J Perinatol. 2019;36(2):124.

35. Aitken K, Cram J, Raymond E, Okun N, Allen L, Windrim R. "Mobile" medicine: a surprise encounter with placenta percreta. J Obstet Gynaecol Can. 2014;36(5):377.
36. Abd Elazeem HAS, Saad MM, Ahmed IA, Sayed EG, AlMahdy AM, Atef F, et al. High-intensity focused ultrasound in management of placenta accreta spectrum: a systematic review. Int J Gynaecol Obstet. 2020;151(3):325–32.
37. Breymann C, Milman N, Mezzacasa A, Bernard R, Dudenhausen J. Ferric carboxymaltose vs. oral iron in the treatment of pregnant women with iron deficiency anemia: an international, open-label, randomized controlled trial (FER-ASAP). J Perinat Med. 2017;45(4):443–53.
38. Tam Tam KB, Dozier J, Martin JN Jr. Approaches to reduce urinary tract injury during management of placenta accreta, increta, and percreta: a systematic review. J Matern Fetal Neonatal Med. 2012;25(4):329–34.
39. Norris BL, Everaerts W, Posma E, Murphy DG, Umstad MP, Costello AJ, et al. The urologist's role in multidisciplinary management of placenta percreta. BJU Int. 2016;117(6):961–5.
40. Wright JD, Silver RM, Bonanno C, Gaddipati S, Lu Y-S, Simpson LL, et al. Practice patterns and knowledge of obstetricians and gynecologists regarding placenta accreta. J Matern Fetal Neonatal Med. 2013;26(16):1602–9.
41. Matsubara S, Kuwata T, Usui R, Watanabe T, Izumi A, Ohkuchi A, et al. Important surgical measures and techniques at cesarean hysterectomy for placenta previa accreta. Acta Obstet Gynecol Scand. 2013;92(4):372–7.
42. Mavrides E, Allard S, Chandraharan E, Collins P, Green L, Hunt B, et al. Prevention and management of postpartum haemorrhage. Am J Obstet Gynecol. 2016;124(5):e106–e49.
43. Green L, Connolly C, Cooper T, Cho G, Allard S. Blood transfusion in obstetrics, guideline no. 47. JLRCoO, Gynaecologists. 2015;
44. Brookfield KF, Goodnough LT, Lyell DJ, Butwick AJ. Perioperative and transfusion outcomes in women undergoing cesarean hysterectomy for abnormal placentation. Transfusion. 2014;54(6):1530–6.
45. Taylor N, Russell R. Anaesthesia for abnormally invasive placenta: a single-institution case series. Int J Obstet Anesth. 2017;30:10–5.
46. Muñoz L, Mendoza G, Gomez M, Reyes L, Arevalo JJ. Anesthetic management of placenta accreta in a low-resource setting: a case series. Int J Obstet Anesth. 2015;24(4):329–34.
47. Kocaoglu N, Gunusen I, Karaman S, Ergenoglu AM, Firat V. Management of anesthesia for cesarean section in parturients with placenta previa with/without placenta accreta: a retrospective study. Ginekol Pol. 2012;83(2)
48. Nguyen Lu N, Carvalho JCA, Windrim R, Allen L, Balki M. Mode of anesthesia and clinical outcomes of patients undergoing Cesarean delivery for invasive placentation: a retrospective cohort study of 50 consecutive cases. Can J Anaesth. 2016;63(11):1233–44.
49. Butwick A, Carvalho B, El-Sayed Y. Risk factors for obstetric morbidity in patients with uterine atony undergoing caesarean delivery. Br J Anaesth. 2014;113(4):661–8.
50. Hong J, Jee Y, Yoon H, Kim S. Comparison of general and epidural anesthesia in elective cesarean section for placenta previa totalis: maternal hemodynamics, blood loss and neonatal outcome. Int J Obstet Anesth. 2003;12(1):12–6.
51. Bratzler DW, Dellinger EP, Olsen KM, Perl TM, Auwaerter PG, Bolon MK, et al. Clinical practice guidelines for antimicrobial prophylaxis in surgery. Am J Health Syst Pharm. 2013;70(3):195–283.
52. Shakur H, Roberts I, Fawole B, Chaudhri R, El-Sheikh M, Akintan A, et al. Effect of early tranexamic acid administration on mortality, hysterectomy, and other morbidities in women with post-partum haemorrhage (WOMAN): an international, randomised, double-blind, placebo-controlled trial. Lancet. 2017;389(10084):2105–16.
53. Sentilhes L, Kayem G, Chandraharan E, Palacios-Jaraquemada J, Jauniaux E, Diagnosis FPA, et al. FIGO consensus guidelines on placenta accreta spectrum disorders: conservative management. Int J Gynaecol Obstet. 2018;140(3):291–8.
54. Woldu SL, Ordonez MA, Devine PC, Wright JD. Urologic considerations of placenta accreta: a contemporary tertiary care institutional experience. Urol Int. 2014;93(1):74–9.

55. Belfort MA, Shamshirsaz AA, Fox KA. A technique to positively identify the vaginal fornices during complicated postpartum hysterectomy. Am J Obstet Gynecol. 2017;217(2):222. e1–3.
56. Camuzcuoglu A, Vural M, Hilali NG, Incebiyik A, Yuce HH, Kucuk A, et al. Surgical management of 58 patients with placenta praevia percreta. Wien Klin Wochenschr. 2016;128(9):360–6.
57. Walker MG, Pollard L, Talati C, Carvalho JC, Allen LM, Kachura J, et al. Obstetric and anaesthesia checklists for the management of morbidly adherent placenta. J Obstet Gynaecol Can. 2016;38(11):1015–23.
58. Jaraquemada JMP, Pesaresi M, Nassif JC, Hermosid S. Anterior placenta percreta: surgical approach, hemostasis and uterine repair. Acta Obstet Gynecol Scand. 2004;83(8):738–44.
59. American College of Obstetricians and Gynecologists. ACOG practice bulletin: clinical management guidelines for obstetrician-gynecologists number 76, October 2006: postpartum hemorrhage. Obstet Gynecol. 2006;108(4):1039–47.
60. Leduc D, Senikas V, Lalonde AB, Ballerman C, Biringer A, Delaney M, et al. Active management of the third stage of labour: prevention and treatment of postpartum hemorrhage. J Obstet Gynaecol Can. 2009;31(10):980–93.
61. Organization WH. WHO recommendations for the prevention and treatment of postpartum haemorrhage: World Health Organization; 2012.
62. Lalonde A, Motherhood FS. Prevention and treatment of postpartum hemorrhage in low-resource settings. Int J Gynaecol Obstet. 2012;117(2):108–18.
63. Sentilhes L, Vayssière C, Deneux-Tharaux C, Aya AG, Bayoumeu F, Bonnet M-P, et al. Postpartum hemorrhage: guidelines for clinical practice from the French College of Gynaecologists and Obstetricians (CNGOF): in collaboration with the French Society of Anesthesiology and Intensive Care (SFAR). Eur J Obstet Gynecol Reprod Biol. 2016;198:12–21.
64. Fitzpatrick K, Sellers S, Spark P, Kurinczuk J, Brocklehurst P, Knight M, et al. The management and outcomes of placenta accreta, increta, and percreta in the UK: a population-based descriptive study. BJOG. 2014;121(1):62–71.
65. Kayem G, Anselem O, Schmitz T, Goffinet F, Davy C, Mignon A, et al. Conservative versus radical management in cases of placenta accreta: a historical study. J Gynecol Obstet Biol Reprod (Paris). 2007;36(7):680–7.
66. Palacios-Jaraquemada J. One-step conservative surgery for abnormal invasive placenta (Placenta Accreta–Increta–Percreta). IJRCOG. 2012:263–71.
67. Palacios-Jaraquemada JM. Diagnosis and management of placenta accreta. Best Pract Res Clin Obstet Gynaecol. 2008;22(6):1133–48.
68. Palacios-Jaraquemada JM. Placental adhesive disorders: Walter de Gruyter; 2012.
69. Chandraharan E, Rao S, Belli A-M, Arulkumaran S. The Triple-P procedure as a conservative surgical alternative to peripartum hysterectomy for placenta percreta. Int J Gynaecol Obstet. 2012;117(2):191–4.
70. Vinas MT, Belli A, Arulkumaran S, Chandraharan E. Prevention of postpartum hemorrhage and hysterectomy in patients with morbidly adherent placenta: a cohort study comparing outcomes before and after introduction of the Triple-P procedure. Ultrasound Obstet Gynecol. 2015;46(3):350–5.
71. Shazly SAE, Badee AY, Ali MK. The use of multiple 8 compression suturing as a novel procedure to preserve fertility in patients with placenta accreta: case series. Aust N Z J Obstet Gynaecol. 2012;52(4):395–9.
72. Huang G, Zhou R, Hu Y. A new suture technique for cesarean delivery complicated by hemorrhage in cases of placenta previa accreta. Int J Gynaecol Obstet. 2014;124(3):262–3.
73. Kaplanoglu M, Kaplanoglu D, Koyuncu O. A different approach to placenta previa accreta: intrauterine gauze compress combined B-Lynch uterine compression suture. Clin Exp Obstet Gynecol. 2015;42(1):53–6.

74. Li GT, Li XF, Li J, Liu YJ, Xu HM. Reflexed compression suture for the management of atonic postpartum hemorrhage with an abnormally adherent placenta. Gynecol Obstet Invest. 2015;80(4):228–33.
75. Li G-T, Li X-F, Wu B, Li GJ. Longitudinal parallel compression suture to control postopartum hemorrhage due to placenta previa and accrete. Gynecol Obstet Invest. 2016;55(2):193–7.
76. El Gelany SA, Abdelraheim AR, Mo'men MM, El-Rab MTG, Yousef AM, Ibrahim EM, et al. The cervix as a natural tamponade in postpartum hemorrhage caused by placenta previa and placenta previa accreta: a prospective study. BMC Pregnancy Childbirth. 2015;15(1):1–7.
77. Allam M, B-Lynch C. The B-Lynch and other uterine compression suture techniques. Int J Gynaecol Obstet. 2005;89(3):236–41.
78. Baskett TF. Uterine compression sutures for postpartum hemorrhage: efficacy, morbidity, and subsequent pregnancy. Obstet Gynecol. 2007;110(1):68–71.
79. Shahin AY, Farghaly TA, Mohamed SA, Shokry M, Abd-El-Aal DEM, Youssef MA. Bilateral uterine artery ligation plus B-lynch procedure for atonic postpartum hemorrhage with placenta accreta. Int J Gynecol Obstet. 2010;108(3):187–90.
80. Doumouchtsis S, Nikolopoulos K, Talaulikar V, Krishna A, Arulkumaran S. Menstrual and fertility outcomes following the surgical management of postpartum haemorrhage: a systematic review. BJOG Int J Obstet Gynaecol. 2014;121(4):382–8.
81. CON-PAS registry. Middle-East Obstetrics and Gynecology Graduate Education (MOGGE) Foundation. https://www.mogge-obgyn.com/con-pas-registry. Last accessed: April 6, 2021.
82. Durukan H, Durukan ÖB, Yazıcı FG. Placenta accreta spectrum disorder: a comparison between fertility-sparing techniques and hysterectomy. J Obstet Gynaecol. 2020:1–7.
83. Bisschop CNS, Schaap TP, Vogelvang TE, Scholten PC. Invasive placentation and uterus preserving treatment modalities: a systematic review. Arch Gynecol Obstet. 2011;284(2):491–502.
84. Sentilhes L, Goffinet F, Kayem G. Management of placenta accreta. Acta Obstet Gynecol Scand. 2013;92(10):1125–34.
85. Sentilhes L, Ambroselli C, Kayem G, Provansal M, Fernandez H, Perrotin F, et al. Maternal outcome after conservative treatment of placenta accreta. Obstet Gynecol. 2010;115(3):526–34.
86. Pather S, Strockyj S, Richards A, Campbell N, de Vries B, Ogle RJA, et al. Maternal outcome after conservative management of placenta percreta at caesarean section: a report of three cases and a review of the literature. Aust N Z J Obstet Gynaecol. 2014;54(1):84–7.
87. Widemann BC, Adamson PC. Understanding and managing methotrexate nephrotoxicity. Oncologist. 2006;11(6):694–703.
88. Lin K, Qin J, Xu K, Hu W, Lin J. Methotrexate management for placenta accreta: a prospective study. Arch Gynecol Obstet. 2015;291(6):1259–64.
89. Isaacs JD Jr, McGehee RP, Cowan BD. Life-threatening neutropenia following methotrexate treatment of ectopic pregnancy: a report of two cases. Obstet Gynecol. 1996;88(4):694–6.
90. Timmermans S, van Hof AC, Duvekot JJ. Conservative management of abnormally invasive placentation. Obstet Gynecol Surv. 2007;62(8):529–39.
91. Mussalli GM, Shah J, Berck DJ, Elimian A, Tejani N, Manning FA. Placenta accreta and methotrexate therapy: three case reports. J Perinatol. 2000;20(5):331–4.
92. Legendre G, Zoulovits FJ, Kinn J, Senthiles L, Fernandez H. Conservative management of placenta accreta: hysteroscopic resection of retained tissues. J Minim Invasive Gynecol. 2014;21(5):910–3.
93. Mazzon I, Favilli A, Grasso M, Horvath S, Gerli S. Is the cold loop hysteroscopic technique a myometrial sparing treatment for placenta accreta residuals in a puerperal uterus? J Matern Fetal Neonatal Med. 2016;29(10):1613–6.
94. Bai Y, Luo X, Li Q, Yin N, Fu X, Zhang H, et al. High-intensity focused ultrasound treatment of placenta accreta after vaginal delivery: a preliminary study. Ultrasound Obstet Gynecol. 2016;47(4):492–8.

95. Jauniaux E, Bhide A. Prenatal ultrasound diagnosis and outcome of placenta previa accreta after cesarean delivery: a systematic review and meta-analysis. Am J Obstet Gynecol. 2017;217(1):27–36.
96. Hudon L, Belfort MA, Broome DR. Diagnosis and management of placenta percreta: a review. Obstet Gynecol Surv. 1999;54(11):156–64.
97. Esakoff TF, Handler SJ, Granados JM, Caughey AB. PAMUS: placenta accreta management across the United States. J Matern Fetal Neonatal Med. 2012;25(6):761–5.
98. Selman AE. Caesarean hysterectomy for placenta praevia/accreta using an approach via the pouch of Douglas. BJOG. 2016;123(5):815–9.
99. Belfort MA, Shamshiraz AA, Fox K. Minimizing blood loss at cesarean-hysterectomy for placenta previa percreta. Am J Obstet Gynecol. 2017;216(1):78. e1–2.
100. Rossetti D, Vitale SG, Bogani G, Rapisarda AMC, Gulino FA, Frigerio L. Usefulness of vessel-sealing devices for peripartum hysterectomy: a retrospective cohort study. Updates Surg. 2015;67(3):301–4.
101. Arendas K, Lortie KJ, Singh SS. Delayed laparoscopic management of placenta increta. J Obstet Gynaecol Can. 2012;34(2):186–9.
102. Smith DD, Perez-Delboy A, Burke WM, Tergas AI. Buttock necrosis after uterine artery embolization for delayed hysterectomy in placenta percreta. Case Rep Obstet Gynecol. 2016;2016:6921280.
103. Rupley DM, Tergas AI, Palmerola KL, Burke WM. Robotically assisted delayed total laparoscopic hysterectomy for placenta percreta. Gynecol Oncol Rep. 2016;17:53–5.
104. Hussein AM, Dakhly DMR, Raslan AN, Kamel A, Abdel Hafeez A, Moussa M, et al. The role of prophylactic internal iliac artery ligation in abnormally invasive placenta undergoing caesarean hysterectomy: a randomized control trial. J Matern Fetal Neonatal Med. (1476–4954 (Electronic)). 2019;32(20):3386–92.
105. Salim R, Chulski A, Romano S, Garmi G, Rudin M, Shalev E, et al. Precesarean prophylactic balloon catheters for suspected placenta accreta: a randomized controlled trial. Obstet Gynecol. 2015;126(5):1022–8.
106. Walker MG, Allen L, Windrim RC, Kachura J, Pollard L, Pantazi S, et al. Multidisciplinary management of invasive placenta previa. J Obstet Gynaecol Can. 2013;35(5):417–25.
107. Sewell MF, Rosenblum D, Ehrenberg H. Arterial embolus during common iliac balloon catheterization at cesarean hysterectomy. Obstet Gynecol. 2006;108(3):746–8.
108. Matsueda S, Hidaka N, Kondo Y, Fujiwara A, Fukushima K. Kato KJJoO, et al. External iliac artery thrombosis after common iliac artery balloon occlusion during cesarean hysterectomy for placenta accreta in cervico-isthmic pregnancy. 2015;41(11):1826–30.
109. Gagnon J, Boucher L, Kaufman I, Brown R, Moore A. Iliac artery rupture related to balloon insertion for placenta accreta causing maternal hemorrhage and neonatal compromise. Can J Anaesth. 2013;60(12):1212–7.
110. Chen L, Wang X, Wang H, Li Q, Shan N, Qi H, et al. Clinical evaluation of prophylactic abdominal aortic balloon occlusion in patients with placenta accreta: a systematic review and meta-analysis. BMC Pregnancy Childbirth. 2019;19(1):1–8.
111. Committee P. Society for Maternal–Fetal Medicine, Belfort MA. Placenta accreta. Am J Obstet Gynecol. 2010;203(5):430–9.
112. Shamshirsaz AA, Carusi D, Shainker SA, Einerson B, Khandelwal M, Erfani H, et al. Characteristics and outcomes of placenta accreta spectrum in twins versus singletons: a study from the pan American Society for Placenta Accreta Spectrum (PAS 2). Am J Obstet Gynecol. 2020;222(6):624–5.
113. Viñas MT, Chandraharan E, Moneta M, Belli A. The role of interventional radiology in reducing haemorrhage and hysterectomy following caesarean section for morbidly adherent placenta. Clin Radiol. 2014;69(8):e345–e51.
114. Bouvier A, Sentilhes L, Thouveny F, Bouet PE, Gillard P, Willoteaux S, et al. Planned caesarean in the interventional radiology cath lab to enable immediate uterine artery embolization for the conservative treatment of placenta accreta. Clin Radiol. 2012;67(11):1089–94.

115. Dilauro MD, Dason S, Athreya S. Prophylactic balloon occlusion of internal iliac arteries in women with placenta accreta: literature review and analysis. Clin Radiol. 2012;67(6):515–20.
116. Clausen C, Stensballe J, Albrechtsen CK, Hansen MA, Lönn L, Langhoff-Roos J. Balloon occlusion of the internal iliac arteries in the multidisciplinary management of placenta percreta. Acta Obstet Gynecol Scand. 2013;92(4):386–91.
117. D'Souza DL, Kingdom JC, Amsalem H, Beecroft JR, Windrim RC, Kachura JR. Conservative management of invasive placenta using combined prophylactic internal iliac artery balloon occlusion and immediate postoperative uterine artery embolization. Can Assoc Radiol J. 2015;66(2):179–84.
118. Chou MM, Kung HF, Hwang JI, Chen WC, Tseng JJ. Temporary prophylactic intravascular balloon occlusion of the common iliac arteries before cesarean hysterectomy for controlling operative blood loss in abnormal placentation. Taiwanese Journal of Obstetrics and Gynecology. 2015;54(5):493–8.
119. Duan XH, Wang YL, Han XW, Chen ZM, Chu QJ, Wang L, et al. Caesarean section combined with temporary aortic balloon occlusion followed by uterine artery embolisation for the management of placenta accreta. Clin Radiol. 2015;70(9):932–7.
120. Wei X, Zhang J, Chu Q, Du Y, Xing N, Xu X, et al. Prophylactic abdominal aorta balloon occlusion during caesarean section: a retrospective case series. Int J Obstet Anesth. 2016;27:3–8.
121. Wu Q, Liu Z, Zhao X, Liu C, Wang Y, Chu Q, et al. Outcome of pregnancies after balloon occlusion of the Infrarenal abdominal aorta during caesarean in 230 patients with placenta Praevia Accreta. Cardiovasc Intervent Radiol. 2016;39(11):1573–9.
122. Xie L, Wang Y, Luo F-Y, Man Y-C, Zhao X-L. Prophylactic use of an infrarenal abdominal aorta balloon catheter in pregnancies complicated by placenta accreta. J Obstet Gynaecol. 2017;37(5):557–61.
123. ACOG committee opinion. Placenta accreta. Number 266, January 2002. American College of Obstetricians and Gynecologists. Int J Gynaecol Obstet. 2002;77(1):77–8.
124. Soyer P, Sirol M, Fargeaudou Y, Bour L, Morel O, Dohan A, et al. Placental vascularity and resorption delay after conservative management of invasive placenta: MR imaging evaluation. Eur Radiol. 2013;23(1):262–71.
125. Organization WH. WHO handbook for guideline development: World Health Organization; 2014.
126. Green S, Pjehl J. Clinical practice guidelines: a guide to better practice, not a recipe for uniformity. Aust J Physiother. 2003;49(1):3–6.
127. Geleris P, Boudoulas H. Problems related to the application of guidelines in clinical practice: a critical analysis. Hell J Cardiol. 2011;52(2):97–102.
128. Wang Z, Norris SL, Bero L. Implementation plans included in World Health Organisation guidelines. Implement Sci. 2015;11(1):1–9.
129. Chong CC. Pros and cons of clinical practice based on guidelines. Hong Kong Med J. 2018;24:440–1.
130. Tinetti ME, Fried T. The end of the disease era. Am J Med. 2004;116(3):179–85.
131. Grol R, Dalhuijsen J, Thomas S, Rutten G, Mokkink H. Attributes of clinical guidelines that influence use of guidelines in general practice: observational study. BMJ. 1998;317(7162):858–61.
132. Shazly SA, Laughlin-Tommaso SK, Dowdy SC, Famuyide AO. Staging for low malignant potential ovarian tumors: a global perspective. Am J Obstet Gynecol. 2016;215(2):153–68. e2.
133. Fox J, Patkar V, Chronakis I, Begent R. From practice guidelines to clinical decision support: closing the loop. J R Soc Med. 2009;102(11):464–73.
134. Flory N, Bissonnette F, Binik YM. Psychosocial effects of hysterectomy: literature review. J Psychosom Res. 2005;59(3):117–29.
135. Naughton MJ, McBee WL. Health-related quality of life after hysterectomy. Clin Obstet Gynecol. 1997;40(4):947–57.

136. Kjerulff KH, Langenberg PW, Rhodes JC, Harvey LA, Guzinski GM, Stolley PD. Effectiveness of hysterectomy. Obstet Gynecol. 2000;95(3):319–26.
137. Marek K, Dimter A, Jawor M, Dudek D. Anxiety-depressive disorders in women after hysterectomy. Literature review. Psychiatria polska. 2001;35(5):763–9.
138. Cal M, Ayres-de-Campos D, Jauniaux E. International survey of practices used in the diagnosis and management of placenta accreta spectrum disorders. Int J Gynaecol Obstet. 2018;140(3):307–11.
139. Jolley JA, Nageotte MP, Wing DA, Shrivastava VK. Management of placenta accreta: a survey of maternal-fetal medicine practitioners. J Matern Fetal Neonatal Med. 2012;25(6):756–60.
140. Matsuzaki S, Yoshino K, Endo M, Kakigano A, Takiuchi T, Kimura T. Conservative management of placenta percreta. Int J Gynaecol Obstet. 2018;140(3):299–306.
141. Mei J, Wang Y, Zou B, Hou Y, Ma T, Chen M, et al. Systematic review of uterus-preserving treatment modalities for abnormally invasive placenta. J Obstet Gynaecol. 2015;35(8):777–82.
142. Steins Bisschop CN, Schaap TP, Vogelvang TE, Scholten PC. Invasive placentation and uterus preserving treatment modalities: a systematic review. Arch Gynecol Obstet. 2011;284(2):491–502.
143. Pinas-Carrillo A, Chandraharan E. Conservative surgical approach: the triple P procedure. Best Pract Res Clin Obstet Gynaecol. 2020;
144. Shmakov RG, Vinitskiy AA, Chuprinin VD, Yarotskaya EL, Sukhikh GT. Alternative approaches to surgical hemostasis in patients with morbidly adherent placenta undergoing fertility-sparing surgery. J Matern Fetal Neonatal Med. 2019;32(12):2042–8.
145. Kallianidis AF, Maraschini A, Danis J, Colmorn LB, Deneux-Tharaux C, Donati S, et al. Epidemiological analysis of peripartum hysterectomy across nine European countries. Acta Obstet Gynecol Scand. 2020;99(10):1364–73.
146. Palacios-Jaraquemada JM, Fiorillo A, Hamer J, Martinez M, Bruno C. Placenta accreta spectrum: a hysterectomy can be prevented in almost 80% of cases using a resective-reconstructive technique. J Matern Fetal Neonatal Med. 2020:1–8.
147. Lional KM, Tagore S, Wright AM. Uterine conservation in placenta accrete spectrum (PAS) disorders: a retrospective case series: is expectant management beneficial in reducing maternal morbidity? Eur J Obstet Gynecol Reprod Biol. 2020;254:212–7.
148. Pather SSS, Richards A, Campbell N, de Vries B, Ogle R. Maternal outcome after conservative management of placenta percreta at caesarean section: a report of three cases and a review of the literature. Aust N Z J Obstet Gynaecol. 2014;54:84–7.
149. Patabendige M, Sanjeewa JMP, Amarasekara AMAKG, Herath RP. Conservative Management of Placenta Percreta: three cases and a review of the literature regarding conservative Management of Placenta Accreta Spectrum (PAS) disorders. Case Rep Obstet Gynecol. 2020;2020:1–7.
150. Bai Y, Luo X, Li Q, Yin N, Fu X, Zhang H, Qi H. High-intensity focused ultrasound treatment of placenta accreta after vaginal delivery: a preliminary study. Ultrasound Obstet Gynecol. 2016;47(4):492–8.
151. Ye M, Yin Z, Xue M, Deng X. High-intensity focused ultrasound combined with hysteroscopic resection for the treatment of placenta accreta. BJOG. 2017;124:71–7.
152. Jiang X, Tang QL, Yang B, Ye F, Cai L, Wang X, Luo X, Bu H. High-intensity focused ultrasound combined procedures treatment of retained placenta accreta with marked vascularity after abortion or delivery. Int J Hyperth. 2019;36(1):421–7.
153. Liu Y, Zhang WW, He M, Gong C, Xie B, Wen X, Li D, Zhang L. Adverse effect analysis of high-intensity focused ultrasound in the treatment of benign uterine diseases. Int J Hyperth. 2018;35(1):56.
154. Palacios-Jaraquemada JM, D'Antonio F, Buca D, Fiorillo A, Larraza P. Systematic review on near miss cases of placenta accreta spectrum disorders: correlation with invasion topography, prenatal imaging, and surgical outcome. J Matern Fetal Neonatal Med. 2020;33(19):3377–84.

Chapter 12
Prevention of Placenta Accreta Spectrum Disorders

Tatiana B. Makukhina and Grigory A. Penzhoyan

Serious complications of placenta accreta spectrum disorders (PAS) for a mother and fetus, the significant risk of hysterectomy with loss of female reproductive function, and expensive hi-tech medical care to patients with this problem attract our attention to clinical research that would promote PAS prevention. Generally speaking, primary prevention aims at reducing the chance of getting the disease, while secondary prophylaxis tries to prevent affected people from deteriorating. *Therefore, primary prevention of PAS* is connected to analysis of risk factors and development of a bundle of measures that would alter modifiable factors.

Primary Prevention of PAS

Restraining the Increase in the Number of CS, Especially in Primiparous

The relationship between expansion of PAS and uprising trend of cesarean section (CS) rates is evident [1–4]. A valuation conducted by Betran AP et al. [5] revealed that CS rate has globally increased from 6.7 % in 1990 to 19.1 % in 2014. A notable growth of CS rate has been linked to extension of indications including caesarean delivery on maternal request (CDMR) [6]. The rate of CDMR differs from country to country; it is difficult to make a comparative estimate as there is no code in the

T. B. Makukhina (✉) · G. A. Penzhoyan
Federal State Budgetary Educational Institution of Higher Education "Kuban State Medical University" of the Ministry of Healthcare of the Russian Federation, Faculty of Postgraduate Education, Department of Obstetrics, Gynecology and Perinatology, Krasnodar, Russia
e-mail: soltatiana@mail.ru

S. A. Shazly, A. A. Nassr (eds.), *Placenta Accreta Spectrum*,
https://doi.org/10.1007/978-3-031-10347-6_12

International Classification of Diseases and discrepancies in that addresses indications of CDMR in the structure of elective CSs [7]. However, approximately 6–8% of all primary CSs were carried out as CDMR in the Great Britain and Northern Europe [8], while in the United States, this figure is 11% [9]. The rate of CDMR in Australia is as high as 17% of all primary CSs [10]. In Germany, some reports indicate that 13% of CSs were performed without medical grounds, although contribution of CDMR to this percentage is not clear [6]. As reported by WHO, the overall annual CS rate in China was 47.6% between 2010 and 2012 [11]. These figures seem to be, at least, constant over time; another prospective study of 3474 primiparous Chinese women demonstrated that prevalence of elective CS was 45.0% between 2012 and 2016. However, relation of these figures to medical indications was not concluded [11]. The social, financial, and cultural factors could be crucial in this equation. In combination with the public misconception that CS is a riskless procedure, private practice could have contributed to the rising prevalence of CS performed [6].

Numerous studies, conducted in different countries, disclose an association between elective CSs and private healthcare facilities in comparison to government-financed facilities, which cannot be merely explained by medical indications [6, 12–15]. Perhaps, there may be a misconception that women who pay for delivery have higher expectations for their own hospital care and the care of their infants than non-paying women. In fact, private practice obstetricians may be more flexible to meet women choices without proper counseling as a sequence of "customer" versus "patient" culture. Interestingly, this may reflect a similar misconception among these obstetricians, who would prefer CS too to ensure a safe delivery. There is some evidence indicating that the probability of an obstetrician to perform CS on maternal request for operative delivery depends more on personal bias, cultural factors, legal liability, and how the request is completed rather than clinical evidence [13]. At the same time, obstetricians may believe in benefits of prelabor CS, such as better control of the delivery process and delivery timing and avoidance of anxiety and necessity of well-trained personnel to monitor labor [7, 13]. In such a way, a randomized controlled trial in a large teaching hospital in Australia appreciated a 22% decrease in CS rate under continuity of midwife-led care compared with birthing under standard care with no difference in perinatal mortality [16].

Interestingly, a relation between rising CS delivery in private clinics and wealth index and household income has been highlighted [12, 15]. Sk R. et al. [15], through an example from India, reported that CS rates were higher among mothers with higher socioeconomic status. The effect of income on CS figures was almost 6.5 times higher than that of delivery setting, whereas most of the income effect was mediated by delivery at private clinics. The rate of elective repeat cesarean delivery (ERCD) in Brazil was higher even in low-risk group, indicating that nonclinical factors may have considerable impact for the decision on CS [17]. More than 80% of women giving birth in public or private health facilities in Brazil wish to have a primary CS, and the rate of CS performed was substantially lower in the public health sector (25% to 30%) than in private clinics (70%) [6]. The assumed effect of private clinics may be more prominent among nulliparous women [13]. This group has a high likelihood of subsequent childbirths and, therefore, the risk of PAS in future pregnancies.

Conducting audits on CS indications is a crucial tool that can potentially control increasing CS rates [14, 18, 19]. According to Lesier E et al. [14], performing audits on CS delivery achieved approximately 2% decline in CS rate. Interventions that aim at implementation of clinical practice guidelines by healthcare professionals combined with mandatory second opinion review of CS indication were associated with slight reduction in overall CS rate (mean difference was –1.9%, 95% CI –3.8 to –0.1). In addition, teaching of physicians by a local opinion former obstetrician-gynecologist decreases the risk of elective CS from 66.8 to 53.7% (opinion former education, 53.7% [95% CI 46.5–61.0]; control, 66.8%, 95% CI 61.7–72.0) [19]. Although the last strategy appears to be the most effective, it may be most beneficial in regions where current CS rates are substantially high, as indicated by the figures in the previous study. Some of these strategies may be more challenging in private practice. Accordingly, parallel patient-centered strategies would be useful to motivate pregnant ladies to undergo normal delivery and correct potential misconceptions. Assessment and correction of the level of anxiety of a pregnant woman could be a promising approach to reduce incidence of CDMRs and prevent PAS in subsequent pregnancies.

Pregnancy-specific anxiety in the second trimester seemed to have a direct impact on CDMR rates among primiparous women [20]. Young pregnant women and women with low level of education are conceivably at high risk of pregnancy-related anxiety [20]. There is another association between CS preference and tokophobia. Risk factors of tokophobia include both anxiety and depression [21]. Indeed, tokophobia is more prevalent than generally perceived, and it ranges between 6 and 10% [22–24]. A survey of 1635 Scandinavian pregnant women revealed that 15.8% and 5.7% had intense and very intense fear of vaginal childbirth, respectively [25], lack of self-confidence in childbirth through vaginal delivery, and unresolved psychosomatic or sexual conflict, which, in combination with the fear of losing control, may also play a part and reinforce the decision to elect for CS [6].

It is necessary to pay attention to maternal psychological problems. Prenatal counseling by medical personnel with appropriate methods should be intensified to defend women against pregnancy-specific anxiety, and the second trimester of pregnancy could be the crucial period for such interventions. Young women and women with a low level of literacy should be the focus groups to conduct the counseling [20].

Psychological education may contribute to spontaneous vaginal delivery rate (relative risk "RR" 1.33, 95% CI 1.11–1.61) [19]. Childbirth classes for single mothers or for couples may decrease incidence of CS (RR 0.55 and 0.59, 95% CI 0.33–0.89 and 0.37–0.94, respectively) and may increase the number of spontaneous vaginal births (RR 2.25 and 2.13, 95% CI 1.16–4.36 and 1.09–4.16, respectively); nursing staff-assisted relaxation training programs and psychosocial prevention programs for couples may reduce CS rate (RR 0.22 and 0.53, 95% CI 0.11–0.43 and 0.32–0.90, respectively) [19]. Joint care by a birth mother and midwife, when the obstetrician provides the birth domiciliary 24 h a day, may provide an alternative to private practices and may reduce primary CS rate [19]. For women having depression during pregnancy, the multidisciplinary approach to patient care and the teamwork of all healthcare providers involved in the process are required to build up supportive environment [21].

The importance of controlling elective CS rate comes from the increased risk of placenta previa and PAS in subsequent pregnancies. This has been confirmed by a number of retrospective design studies: case-control study (odds ratio (OR) 3.00; 95% CI 1.47–6.12) [26]; case-control study (OR 3.32; 95% CI 1.68–6.58) [27]; retrospective cohort study of 8208 women (adjusted odds ratio [aOR] 2.52; 95% CI 1.53–4.14) [28]; retrospective cohort study of 26,987 women (aOR 2.62; 95% CI 1.24–5.56) [29], and prospective cohort study of 34,224 women (aOR 2.03; 95% CI 1.22–3.38) [30]. There are some data that propose a causal relation between uterine damage and uterine incision level, where a more caudal incision would be associated with uterine damage [31]. Subsequently, Matsubara S. et al. hypothesized that the timing of elective CS should ideally be performed after onset of labor. Obviously, the authors addressed subsequent risks of emergency and uncontrolled CSs, which are associated with worse outcomes compared to elective CS. Alternative, the authors proposed controlled oxytocin administration prior to elective CS to induce labor-positive status [31]. Unfortunately, this practice cannot be recommended as a routine measure to prevent PAS in a subsequent pregnancy. There is no definitive protocol or duration of oxytocin administration that would be deemed sufficient to provide a significant reduction in uterine damage and PAS risk in subsequent pregnancy. Since uterine response is variable, such protocol is challenging to be determined. In addition, given the low incidence of PAS, assessment of oxytocin impact would require a large sample size, and likely many women would be unnecessarily exposed to oxytocin for a single patient, if any, to benefit from this approach. Furthermore, use of oxytocin is not without risk, and it may result in fetal distress. Administration-to-action would be variable and exact time of fasting and procedure would be hard to schedule. In fact, Zeevi G et al., in a population-based retrospective cohort study, have not revealed a difference in frequency of subsequent PAS depending on whether the patient had CS before the onset of labor or in the active phase of labor. On the contrary, risk of complications due to PAS would be significantly higher in the case of emergency CS [32].

In summary, the most likely effective measurement for PAS prevention is counseling, education, and psychological support. This includes counseling women who opt for CDMR on possible complications on subsequent pregnancy, including the chance of abnormal placement (placenta previa OR 1.74 [95% CI 1.62–1.87], accreta OR 2.95 [95% CI = 1.32–6.60], and abruption (OR 1.38 [95% CI 1.27–1.49]) [33]. This approach has been supported by several national guidelines [2, 7].

Orientation of Pregnant Women with a Scar on the Uterus After CS to Attempt Vaginal Delivery in the Absence of Other Indications for CS

Repeat CSs are one of the most evident risk factors of PAS in subsequent pregnancies, and incidence of PAS is directly proportional to a number of previous CSs [34]. Specifically, women who had one, two, and three prior cesarean deliveries were 2.9, 4.6, and 12.6 times most probably to have PAS, respectively [34]. Therefore, efforts to reduce incidence of PAS should include women with previous CS and their plan for delivery. Vaginal birth after CS (VBAC) does not only reduce incidence of PAS in subsequent pregnancies but also precludes complications associated with repeated abdominal surgeries such as hysterectomy, bladder or bowel injury, and massive blood loss requiring blood transfusion and reduces risk of related infection [35]. Thus, VBAC has been widely supported by the National Institute for Health and Care Excellence (NICE), Royal College of Obstetricians and Gynaecologists (RCOG), and American College of Obstetricians and Gynecologists (ACOG) as a clinically safe and recommended approach for majority of women who had a single previous lower segment CS [36]. This strategy is also backed up by the health economic modeling and would also at least restrict potential rise in CS and maternal morbidity associated with repeated surgeries [36]. Based on statistical reports from different countries, up to 50% of patients with previous CS scar are eligible to attempt vaginal delivery [37–39].

Nevertheless, the potential of this practice in controlling number of repeated CSs is not used in full. In the United Kingdom, the rate of trial of labor after cesarean delivery (TOLAC), according to a cohort study involving 143,970 women, was 75,086 (52.2%), and 47,602 women (63.4%) successfully achieved vaginal delivery [40]. In China, the rate of VBAC after relaxation of the one-child policy in 2013 was 9.8% [11], while in the United States, the rate of VBAC dropped from 28.3% in 1996 to 8.5% in 2006 [35]. Between January 2013 and December 2015, 34,460 women, from the Japanese nationwide institution-based registry, were investigated. Only 1730 (5.0%) underwent TOLAC versus 32,730 (95.0%) who had ERCD, respectively. Approximately 76% of clinics did not perform any TOLACs. On the other hand, most women (88.6%), attempting TOLAC, had successful vaginal deliveries [41]. Data from case series of women attempting TOLAC demonstrated that 52–82% achieve vaginal delivery [35, 42–44]. There is probably no single explanation to the discrepancy in TOLAC rates worldwide. However, magnitude of contribution of private sector versus governmental services in medical care and strict oversight of rates of CS may play a role.

Nevertheless, thoughtful selection of candidates for VBAC is crucial, since risk of maternal morbidity is related to a woman's probability of achieving VBAC [35]. Most maternal TOLAC- related complications arise when intrapartum repeat cesarean delivery is required. In view of this, VBAC is associated with fewer complications than ERCD, while an unsuccessful TOLAC yields the highest risk of complications [35]. Probability of successful VBAC varies, depending on women demographic and obstetric characteristics, and is a subject to individual combination of antepartum and intrapartum factors. There are scoring systems and calculators that assist in predicting probability of VBAC success [35]. ACOG suggests that a probability above 70% would support TOLAC over ERCD, while a probability below 60% would favor ERCD. A percentage between 60% and 70% is indeterminate, and risks vs. benefits of both options are considered balanced [35]. This information is commonly considered for patient counseling. Although there are no standard cutoff probabilities that would contraindicate vaginal delivery, many institutes adopt internal policies that do not offer TOLAC if calculated score is below a certain percentage. On the contrary, the RCOG [36] adopted planned VBAC, which can be offered to majority of women with after a single previous lower segment caesarean delivery, with or without a history of previous vaginal birth. VBAC probability scores are not adopted by RCOG, and TOLAC is offered universally to all eligible women [36]. This could present another factor that would contribute to broader TOLAC practice in the United Kingdom.

ACOG recommendations [35] related to two previous low-transverse cesarean scars, and twin pregnancy, and breech presentation including external cephalic version (in women having one previous cesarean delivery with a low-transverse incision) do not consider these conditions as contraindications to TOLAC. RCOG [36] also does not preclude the possibility of TOLAC for patients with two scars after CS. However, it highlights that risk of uterine rupture would be higher in this population and, accordingly, the decision should be made with caution in highly motivated women and is unlikely to include induction of labor as a part of TOLAC. Obstetricians should be aware of cultural backgrounds and family planning decision, when leading a counseling discussion, since some couples may be highly motivated to have many children as opposed to those who opt for two to three children. As mentioned earlier, the dose-response relationship documented between placenta accreta and the number of prior CSs, especially in the setting of placenta previa, should always be considered [45].

A woman's desire for TOLAC is an extremely determining factor in VBAC prevalence. ACOG [35] encourages obstetricians to thoroughly discuss both potential risks and benefits of TOLAC and ERCD and to document these discussions. Discussing VBAC early, during a woman's prenatal care course, will give more time for her to analyze both options and bring more questions and concerns. Also, further research on information gaps reported by women, and their impact on decision-making, would be of great benefit [46–48]. In addition, medical sector should be readily supported to achieve more VBACs. The high rate of ERCD in private clinics suggests that one of the many factors contributing to this trend is that the medical personnel of private clinics are not motivated to convince the CDMR-oriented patients of vaginal delivery. For instance, in the private sector of Brazil, almost all deliveries (95.8%) were performed by ERCD as compared with 44.1% in the public sector ($p < 0{,}001$) [17]. Meanwhile, ERCD in the public sector was related to social and economic (better education), obstetric (women's preference, absence of previous vaginal delivery, macrosomia), and hospital (mixed hospital, location in non-capital city, less than 1500 deliveries per year) characteristics [17]. Accordingly, alternative strategies should be proposed to incorporate private practice in the ongoing efforts to reduce CS rates and provide support and utilities to ensure VBAC practice would be supported.

Thus, the strategy for reducing the risk of PAS is a set of measures aimed at reducing the number of elective CS in both primiparous women and women with a scar on the uterus after CS. This is possible with the availability of psychological, specialized medical care for a pregnant woman, beginning from the first trimester of pregnancy, to form a dominant for a successful vaginal delivery in the absence of medical indications for CS. Also, probability of vaginal delivery is higher in the case of a patient's delivery in a large public hospital, with the possibility of monitoring by qualified personnel. A small number of interventions, mainly targeting healthcare specialists (such as introduction of guidelines, mandatory second opinion, constant audit and feedback, training of physicians by a local opinion former) have been shown to safely reduce caesarean section rates [19].

The Guideline Development Group of the World Health Organization (WHO) presented recommendations for nonclinical interventions to reduce CS births [49]. These recommendations are classified based on the purpose of the intervention: (a) interventions intended for women, (b) interventions intended for healthcare specialists, and (c) interventions intended for organizations, institutions, or health systems. The WHO recommends the use of various educational programs for women in the process of their preparation for childbirth to reduce the number of caesarean sections. However, this recommendation has a low-certainty evidence [49].

Modifying Other PAS-Related Risk Factors

Placenta Previa (PP)

Women with PP were 34.9 times highly likely to have placenta accreta than those women without previa (95% CI 2.4–54.3) [34]. In the view of some experts, this pathology is a type of PAS (PAS 0) [50]. PP and PAS risk factors largely overlap. According to Gargari S et al. [51], maternal age, multiparity, history of stillbirth, history of dilatation and evacuation, and history of CS increase the risk of PP in subsequent pregnancy (aOR 2.02, 95% CI 1.35–3.05) [28]. Although there are no prevention strategies for PP, strategies to reduce CS rates would be the most crucial since PAS risk is most prominent when PP is associated with uterine scar.

Previous Uterine Surgery

Uterine surgeries, other than CS, also contribute to PAS risk [4]. Similar to CS, these surgeries precipitate focal loss of endometrium and myometrium, and this effect may be more prominent if performed during pregnancy. Minor uterine surgeries (i.e., dilatation and curettage, hysteroscopic surgery), particularly if performed more than three times, were associated with higher probability of PAS in subsequent pregnancies (OR 3.4; 95% CI 1.3–8.9) [52]. Similar to CS, the relationship between number of other uterine procedures and development of PAS is "dose-dependent" [53]. Procedures that may impact integrity of the uterine mucosa like manual delivery of the placenta, postpartum endometritis, and uterine artery embolization have been considered as risk factors for PAS [1]. Yang T. et al. [54] describe the history of myomectomy as a risk factor for PAS, but not as an independent one. O'Malley KN et al. [30] did not find a significant increase in the risk of PAS after the preceding myomectomy in a cohort that included more than 34,000 observations of patients with a history of CS. Nevertheless, information on the sequence of myomectomy and the first CS was not available in this study. March CM investigated the outcomes of 1240 infertile women treated for intrauterine adhesions and reported 13 (2%) cases of PAS in subsequent pregnancies [55].

However, with due regard to the prevalence of surgical interventions on the uterus in comparison to incidence of PAS, it seems unlikely that significant reduction in incidence of PAS would be achieved by preventing surgeries, a significant part of which aims at restoring fertility or managing an urgent obstetric complication. Rather, a cautious approach should be taken to assess risk of PAS among women with previous uterine surgeries when planning pregnancy, including conscious first trimester assessment for early suspicion and secondary prevention. Obstetricians and midwives should take proper history to identify these surgeries specially when medical records are not available [56, 57].

Advanced Maternal Age

Maternal age of 35 years or older has been a suggested risk factor of PAS. A Scandinavian cohort study of 605,567 women found that advance maternal age was associated with increased risk of PAS (OR 4.6; 95% CI 3.2–6.7). However, this association may be prone to several confounders, rather than with isolated maternal age [4]. This relationship may be hindered by impact of age on parity, increased number of CSs, higher risk of PP, as well as a higher likelihood of preceding uterine surgeries or fertility medical procedure but also may represent an altered hormonal or implantation environment [34, 54, 56, 57]. In fact, a multivariable logistic regression conducted by Bowman ZS et al. did not find significant association between maternal age greater than 40 years and parity, hypertension, diabetes, race, pre-pregnancy body mass index, education, and risk of PAS [34].

Regardless, pregnancy at age 35 or older does not typically present a modifiable risk factor of PAS and cannot be used in the structure of preventive measures directly. However, this information may be indirectly used during preconception counseling and reproductive decision-making when couples consider their plans [56].

Interpregnancy Interval

Yang T. et al. [54] endorsed significant difference in incidence of PAS in patients with longer intervals between the last CS and current pregnancy from 71.78 to 91.14 months ($p < 0.001$). However, when adjusted for other confounders, Bowman. et al. [34] did not appreciate significant risk in relation to this variable. Thus, the possibility of using the interpregnancy interval to reduce the likelihood of developing PAS requires further study.

Smoking

Generally, smoking is associated with increased risk of several medical, obstetric, and perinatal complications, including PP and stillbirth [2, 58]. Although there is no robust evidence that smoking solely increases risk of PAS [34], smoking session is an integral part of preconception and antenatal care and should always be encouraged [59].

CS Technique

The rising rates of PAS in the current century may not be only contributed to substantial increase in CS rates. Interestingly, incidence of PAS has doubled among women with previous CS scars since 2000, suggesting potential contribution of other surgical factors to this incidence [60]. One theory attributed this trend possibly to the change in suture material, which may alter uterine ability to heal after surgery and predispose to trophoblastic invasion in subsequent pregnancies [60]. Practice change related to peritoneal closure may have contributed at a time since now there is growing evidence that peritoneal closure does not reduce adhesion formation and it may increase risk of infectious and febrile morbidity [61]. Obviously, these theories attempt to find a causal relation between change in practice and healing process since the quality of uterine scar directly impacts the pathophysiology of PAS [62].

Consequently, parallel directions have been investigated to identify technical strategies that would reduce deficient uterine healing and probability of PAS in subsequent pregnancies. Sumigama S et al. investigated the impact of suturing technique on PAS incidence, and their results showed that hysterotomy closure using interrupted sutures was associated with lower probability of future PAS compared to continuous suturing [63]. Nevertheless, a meta-analysis of nine randomized controlled trials, including 3696 participants, concluded that the number of layers does not strongly influence uterine scar healing and that there was no significant difference in uterine scar defects when single-layer was compared to double-layer closure (RR 0.77, 95% CI 0.36–1.64) [64]. Two more recent randomized controlled trials reported that double-layer closure with unlocked first layer was associated with better uterine scar healing as compared to locked single layer. However, this study assessed residual myometrial thickness as an indicator of healing, but not incidence of PAS in subsequent pregnancy [65, 66]. Another prospective study investigated possible risk factors of niche formation after CS and found no difference in outcomes depending on the urgency of CS indication. Most contributing factors were gestational diabetes (OR 1.73; 95% CI 1.02–2.92), previous cesarean delivery (OR 3.14; 95% CI 1.90–5.17), and higher maternal body mass index (OR 1.06; 95% CI 1.01–1.11). Surgical techniques were not studied. Again, this study indirectly investigated CS healing process, but not the risk of PAS [67]. There is currently insufficient evidence to support interpregnancy correction or cesarean scar revision with different surgical techniques [68].

With due regard to difficulties in the comparative assessment of the probability of the impact of this factor on the formation of PAS in subsequent pregnancy, the problem requires further study. It can be assumed that subsequent studies will be aimed not only at determining the benefits of various surgical techniques but also at using biological agents that improve tissue healing. Modification of this risk factor at the current stage of our understanding of the development of pathology has no practical significance.

Assisted Reproductive Technologies

These technologies increase the risk of PAS approximately three times (OR 3.1; 95% CI = 1.6–5.8) [57]. Some studies have shown that cryopreserved embryo transfer has a higher risk for PAS, retained placenta, and postpartum hemorrhage than a fresh in vitro fertilization cycle [69, 70]. Kaser DJ et al. [71] showed that PAS was associated with a significantly thinner preimplantation endometrium, which occurs in unstimulated cryopreserved embryo transfer cycles with uterine preparation. Further research is warranted to distinguish the direct role of embryo freezing from related endometrial factors and to determine potential modifiable risk factors for abnormal placentation, such as method of freezing or endometrial preparation [72].

In summary, strategies of primary prevention of PAS should be based on the public education national policy, focused on modifying numerous additional PAS risk factors: formation of a dominant for the timely implementation of fertility, prevention of unplanned pregnancy, smoking cessation, etc. Further studies on the impact of potentially causative factors that would increase the risk of PAS from the standpoints of evidence-based medicine are needed.

Secondary Prevention of PAS

Secondary prevention of PAS intends to prevent complications, which would be associated with significant morbidity, mortality, and adverse reproductive outcomes. A cornerstone to achieve secondary prevention is to promote early diagnosis of PAS. Numerous medical communities including the International Federation of Gynecology and Obstetrics (FIGO), Society for Maternal-Fetal Medicine (SMFM), ACOG, RCOG, and Society of Obstetricians and Gynaecologists of Canada (SOGC) emphasize on the possibility of suspecting and diagnosing PAS in the first trimester [2–4, 73, 74]. Many experts use the term "caesarean scar pregnancy" (CSP) to refer to abnormal invasion in the first trimester, specifying that CSP and PAS are stages of a single process of abnormal invasion of placenta [75–80]. With due regard to high risks of CSP progression, experts of FIGO, SCOG, and SMFM recommend pregnancy termination as soon as the diagnosis is confirmed, a strategy that can be considered as secondary prevention of PAS [4, 68, 73].

Challenges to secondary prevention include lack of robust sonographic indicators of risk and degree of PAS in asymptomatic patients particularly early in pregnancy [2, 76, 80, 81]. Determination of reliable predictive criteria is hindered by small sample sizes, retrospective designs of most studies investigating early ultrasound diagnosis of PAS, and wide variation in definition and inclusion criteria, which leads to inconsistency in performance and skewed sensitivity [72, 76, 78, 82–84].

Feasibility of early ultrasound scan at 5–8 weeks of pregnancy to identify implantation site of gestation sac is approved by many experts [80, 85]. Nevertheless, introduction of mandatory early ultrasound scans for the purpose of early PAS diagnosis in patients with CS scars was investigated in Italy, and it has not contributed to lowering PAS rate [86]. Thus, further investigations are required to optimize and validate the value of this strategy.

Studying biochemical markers of abnormal placentation is another approach that yields promising results. Many studies linked elevated PAPP-A and β-hCG to PAS in the first trimester [87–90]. However, these markers are nonspecific, and they have been associated with a variety of maternal and fetal conditions. Therefore, interpretation of results should be carefully made in concordance with clinical background. Currently, there is insufficient evidence to recommend utilization of first trimester maternal serum level of biomarkers to screen for PAS disorders, and further investigations are merited [4, 73].

Future research should consider developing robust prediction models that could stratify risk early and differentiate women at higher risk of first-trimester symptoms from those in which progression to viability, although potentially complicated by PAS disorders, is more likely [73, 80]. Standardization of available data and identification of additional informative features are necessary for development of a model of contingent screening in the first trimester of pregnancy. Such screening could combine sonographic, biochemical marker, and clinical information to identify PAS risk. Contingent screening in the first trimester could present the basis of secondary prevention. In addition, early diagnosis and routing to comprehensive care in a specialized center are critical to reduce maternal morbidity and mortality.

References

1. Jauniaux E, Chantraine F, Silver RM, Langhoff-Ross J. For the FIGO placenta accreta diagnosis and management expert consensus panel. FIGO consensus guidelines on placenta accreta spectrum disorders: epidemiology. Int J Gynecol Obstet. 2018;140:265e73.
2. Jauniaux ERM, Alfirevic Z, Bhide AG, Belfort MA, Burton GJ, Collins SL, et al. Placenta praevia and placenta accreta: diagnosis and management. Green-top guideline no. 27a. BJOG. 2018;
3. Cahill AG, Beigi R, Heine RP, Silver RM, Wax JR. Placenta accreta spectrum. Practice guideline. Am J Obstet Gynecol. 2018;219(6):B2–B16. https://doi.org/10.1016/j.ajog.2018.09.042. ACOG
4. SOGC clinical practice guideline No. 383. Screening, diagnosis, and management of placenta accreta spectrum disorders. J Obstet Gynaecol Can. 2019;41(7):1035–49. https://doi.org/10.1016/j.jogc.2018.12.004.
5. Betran AP, Ye J, Moller A-B, Zhang J, Gulmezoglu AM, Torloni MR. The increasing trend in caesarean section rates: global, regional and National Estimates: 1990–2014. PLoS One [Internet]. 2016;11(2):e0148343. Available from: http://www.pubmedcentral.nih.gov/articlerender.fcgi?artid=4743929&tool=pmcentrez&rendertype=abstract
6. Mylonas I, Friese K. The indications for and risks of elective CS. Dtsch Arztebl Int. 2015;112:489–95. https://doi.org/10.3238/arztebl.2015.0489.
7. Alsayegh E, Bos H, Campbell K, Barrett J. Caesarean delivery on maternal request. Practice guideline no. 361. J Obstet Gynaecol Can. 2018;40(7):967–71. https://doi.org/10.1016/j.jogc.2017.12.009.
8. National Institute for Health and Clinical Excellence: Caesarean Section. NICE clinical guideline №132. 2nd ed. RCOG Press; 2011.
9. MacDorman M, Declercq E, Menacker F. Recent trends and patterns in cesarean and vaginal birth after cesarean (VBAC) deliveries in the United States. Clin Perinatol. 2011;38:179–92.
10. Robson SJ, Tan WS, Adeyemi A, Dear KB. Estimating the rate of CS by maternal request: anonymous survey of obstetricians in Australia. Birth. 2009;36:208–12.
11. Mu Y, Li X, Zhu J, Liu Z, Li M, Deng K, Deng C, Li Q, Kang L, Wang Y, Liang J. Prior caesarean section and likelihood of vaginal birth, 2012-2016, China. Bull World Health Organ. 2018;96(8):548–57. https://doi.org/10.2471/BLT.17.206433.
12. Kambale MJ. Social predictors of caesarean section births in Italy. Afr Health Sci. 2012;11(4):560–5.
13. Einarsdóttir K, Haggar F, Pereira G, et al. Role of public and private funding in the rising caesarean section rate: a cohort study. BMJ Open. 2013;3:e002789. https://doi.org/10.1136/bmjopen-2013-002789.
14. Lesieur E, Blanc J, Loundou A, Claquin A, Marcot M, Heckenroth H, et al. Teaching and performing audits on caesarean delivery reduce the caesarean delivery rate. PLoS One. 2018;13(8):e0202475. https://doi.org/10.1371/journal.pone.0202475.
15. Sk R. Does delivery in private hospitals contribute largely to caesarean section births? A path analysis using generalised structural equation modelling. PLoS One. 2020;15(10):e0239649. https://doi.org/10.1371/journal.pone.0239649.
16. McLachlan H, Forster D, Davey M, et al. Effects of continuity of care by a primary midwife (caseload midwifery) on caesarean section rates in women of low obstetric risk: the COSMOS randomised controlled trial. BJOG. 2012;119:1483–92.
17. Nakamura-Pereira M, Esteves-Pereira AP, Gama SGN, Leal M. Elective repeat cesarean delivery in women eligible for trial of labor in Brazil. Int J Gynaecol Obstet. 2018;143(3):351–9. https://doi.org/10.1002/ijgo.12660.
18. Paracchini S, Masturzo B, Tangolo D, Roletti E, Piazzese A, Attini R, Rolfo A, Todros T. Upcoming strategies in obstetrics: how the technology of clinical audit may reduce cesarean birth. Minerva Ginecol. 2017;69(6):548–54. https://doi.org/10.23736/S0026-4784.17.04035-7.

19. Chen I, Opiyo N, Tavender E, Mortazhejri S, Rader T, Petkovic J, Yogasingam S, Taljaard M, Agarwal S, Laopaiboon M, Wasiak J, Khunpradit S, Lumbiganon P, Gruen RL, Betran AP. Non-clinical interventions for reducing unnecessary caesarean section. Cochrane Database Syst Rev. 2018;9(9):CD005528. https://doi.org/10.1002/14651858.CD005528.pub3.
20. Sun Y, Huang K, Hu Y, Yan S, Xu Y, Zhu P, et al. Pregnancy-specific anxiety and elective CS in primiparas: A cohort study in China. PLoS One. 2019;14(5):e0216870. https://doi.org/10.1371/journal.pone.0216870.
21. Demšar K, Svetina M, Verdenik I, Tul N, Blickstein I, Globevnik VV. Tokophobia (fear of childbirth): prevalence and risk factors. J Perinat Med. 2018;46(2):151–4. https://doi.org/10.1515/jpm-2016-0282.
22. Wiklund I, Edman G, Andolf E. CS on maternal request: reasons for the request, self-estimated health, expectations, experience of birth and signs of depression among first-time mothers. Acta Obstet Gynecol Scand. 2007;86:451–6.
23. Wiklund I. New guidelines for CS on maternal request. Sex Reprod Healthc. 2012;3:97.
24. Sahlin M, Carlander-Klint AK, Hildingsson I, Wiklund I. First-time mothers' wish for a planned caesarean section: deeply rooted emotions. Midwifery. 2013;29:447–52.
25. Nieminen K, Stephansson O, Ryding EL. Women's fear of childbirth and preference for CS–a cross-sectional study at various stages of pregnancy in Sweden. Acta Obstet Gynecol Scand. 2009;88:807–13.
26. Kamara M, Henderson JJ, Doherty DA, et al. The risk of placenta accreta following primary elective caesarean delivery: a case-control study. BJOG. 2013;120:879–86.
27. Shi XM, Wang Y, Zhang Y, Wei Y, Chen L, Zhao YY, et al. Effect of primary elective cesarean delivery on placenta accreta: A case-control study. Chin Med J. 2018;131:672–6. https://doi.org/10.4103/0366-6999.226902.
28. Chen S, Cheng W, Chen Y, Liu X. The risk of abnormal placentation and hemorrhage in subsequent pregnancy following primary elective cesarean delivery. J Matern Fetal Neonatal Med. 2020;33(21):3608–13. https://doi.org/10.1080/14767058.2019.1581167. Epub 2019 Feb 27
29. Downes KL, Hinkle SN, Sjaarda LA, Albert PS, Grantz KL. Previous prelabor or intrapartum cesarean delivery and risk of placenta previa. Am J Obstet Gynecol. 2015;212(5):669.e1–6. https://doi.org/10.1016/j.ajog.2015.01.004. Epub 2015 Jan 7
30. O'Malley KN, Norton ME, Osmundson SS. Effect of trial of labor before cesarean and risk of subsequent placenta Accreta Spectrum disorders. Am J Perinatol. 2020;37(6):633–7. https://doi.org/10.1055/s-0039-1685449. Epub 2019 Apr 16
31. Matsubara S, Takahashi H. Placenta Previa Accreta and previous CS: some clarifications. Chin Med J (Engl). 2018;131(12):1504–5. https://doi.org/10.4103/0366-6999.233961.
32. Zeevi G, Tirosh D, Baron J, Sade MY, Segal A, Hershkovitz R. The risk of placenta accreta following primary cesarean delivery. Arch Gynecol Obstet. 2018;297(5):1151–6. https://doi.org/10.1007/s00404-018-4698-4. Epub 2018 Feb 5
33. Keag OE, Norman JE, Stock SJ. Long-term risks and benefits associated with cesarean delivery for mother, baby, and subsequent pregnancies: systematic review and meta-analysis. PLoS Med. 2018;15(1)
34. Bowman ZS, Eller AG, Bardsley TR, Greene T, Varner MW, Silver RM. Risk factors for placenta accreta: a large prospective cohort. Am J Perinatol. 2014;31:799–804. https://doi.org/10.1055/s-0033-1361833.
35. ACOG Practice Bulletin No. 205. Vaginal birth after cesarean delivery. Obstetrics&Gynecology. 2019;133(2):e110–27. https://doi.org/10.1097/AOG.0000000000003078.
36. Birth After Previous Caesarean Birth (2015). RCOG Green-top Guideline No 45.
37. Hamilton B, Martin J, Osterman M, Driscoll A, Rossen L. Births: provisional data for 2016. Vital statistics rapid release no 2. Hyattsville (MD): National Center for Health Statistics; 2017.
38. Dodd JM, Crowther CA, Huertas E, Guise J-M, Horey D. Planned elective repeat caesarean section versus planned vaginal birth for women with a previous caesarean birth. Cochrane Database Syst Rev. 2013;12:CD004224.

39. Little MO, Lyerly AD, Mitchell LM, Armstrong EM, Harris LH, Kukla R, et al. Mode of delivery: toward responsible inclusion of patient preferences. Obstet Gynecol. 2008;112(4):913–8.
40. Knight HE, Gurol-Urganci I, van der Meulen JH, Mahmood TA, Richmond DH, Dougall A, Cromwell DA. Vaginal birth after caesarean section: a cohort study investigating factors associated with its uptake and success. BJOG. 2014;121(2):183–92. https://doi.org/10.1111/1471-0528.12508. Epub 2013 Nov 20
41. Takeya A, Adachi E, Takahashi Y, Kondoh E, Mandai M, Nakayama T. Trial of labor after cesarean delivery (TOLAC) in Japan: rates and complications. Arch Gynecol Obstet. 2020;301(4):995–1001. https://doi.org/10.1007/s00404-020-05492-8. Epub 2020 Mar 17
42. Gobillot S, Ghenassia A, Coston AL, Gillois P, Equy V, Michy T, Hoffmann P. Obstetric outcomes associated with induction of labour after caesarean section. J Gynecol Obstet Hum Reprod. 2018;47(10):539–43. https://doi.org/10.1016/j.jogoh.2018.09.006. Epub 2018 Sep 22
43. Li Y-X, Bai Z, Long D-J, Wang H-B, Wu Y-F, Reilly KH, Huang S-R, Ji Y-J. Predicting the success of vaginal birth after caesarean delivery: a retrospective cohort study in China. Multicenter Study BMJ Open. 2019;9(5):e027807. https://doi.org/10.1136/bmjopen-2018-027807.
44. Vuchenovich YD, Novikova VA, Radzinsky VE. An alternative to repeat CS. Doctor. 2020;19(6):15–22. https://doi.org/10.31550/1727-2378-2020-19-6-15-22.
45. Silver RM, Landon MB, Rouse DJ, et al. National Institute of child health and human development maternal-fetal medicine units network. Maternal morbidity associated with multiple repeat cesarean deliveries. Obstet Gynecol. 2006;107:1226–32.
46. Nilsson C, Lalor J, Begley C, Carroll M, Gross MM, Grylka-Baeschlin S, Lundgren I, Matterne A, Morano S, Nicoletti J, Healy P. Vaginal birth after caesarean: views of women from countries with low VBAC rates. Women Birth. 2017;30(6):481–90. https://doi.org/10.1016/j.wombi.2017.04.009.
47. Lundgren I, Morano S, Nilsson C, Sinclair M, Begley C. Cultural perspectives on vaginal birth after previous caesarean section in countries with high and low rates - A hermeneutic study. Women Birth. 2020;33(4):e339–47. https://doi.org/10.1016/j.wombi.2019.07.300.
48. Rietveld AL, van Exel NJA, Cohen de Lara MC, de Groot CJM, Teunissen PW. Giving birth after caesarean: identifying shared preferences among pregnant women using Q methodology. Women Birth. 2020;33(3):273–9. https://doi.org/10.1016/j.wombi.2019.05.005.
49. WHO recommendations non-clinical interventions to reduce unnecessary caesarean sections. (2018). Geneva: World Health Organization; Licence: CC BY-NC-SA 3.0 IGO. Cataloguing-in-Publication (CIP) data. CIP data are available at http://apps.who.int/iris.
50. Cali G, Forlani F, Lees C, Timor-Tritsch I, Palacios-Jaraquemada J, Dall'Asta A, Bhide A, Flacco ME, Manzoli L, Labate F, Perino A, Scambia G, D'Antonio F. Prenatal ultrasound staging system for placenta accrete spectrum disorders. Ultrasound Obstet Gynecol. 2019;53:752–60. https://doi.org/10.1002/uog.20246.
51. Gargari Saleh S, Seify Z, Haghighi L, Khoshnood Shariati M, Mirzamoradi M. Risk factors and consequent outcomes of placenta Previa: report from a referral center. Acta Med Iran. 2016;54(11):713–7.
52. Fitzpatrick KE, Sellers S, Spark P, et al. Incidence and risk factors for placenta accreta/increta/percreta in the UK: a national case-control study. PLoS One. 2012;7:e52893.
53. Baldwin HJ, Patterson JA, Nippita TA, et al. Antecedents of abnormally invasive placenta in primiparous women: risk associated with gynecologic procedures. Obstet Gynecol. 2018;131:227–33.
54. Yang T, Li N, Qiao C, Liu C. Development of a novel nomogram for predicting placenta Accreta in patients with scarred uterus: A retrospective cohort study. Front Med. 2019;6:289. https://doi.org/10.3389/fmed.2019.00289.
55. March CM. Asherman's syndrome. Semin Reprod Med. 2011;29(2):83–94. https://doi.org/10.1055/s-0031-1272470. Epub 2011 Mar 24
56. Carusi DA. The placenta Accreta Spectrum: epidemiology and risk factors. Clinical Obstet Gynecol. 2018;00(00). www.clinicalobgyn.com

57. Thurn L, Lindqvist PG, Jakobsson M, Colmorn LB, Klungsoyr K, Bjarnadóttir RI, Tapper AM, Børdahl PE, Gottvall K, Petersen KB, Krebs L, Gissler M, Langhoff-Roos J, Källen K. Abnormally invasive placentaprevalence, risk factors and antenatal suspicion: results from a large population-based pregnancy cohort study in the Nordic countries. BJOG. 2016;123:1348–55. https://doi.org/10.1111/1471-0528.13547.
58. Management of Stillbirth: Obstetric Care Consensus No, 10. SMFM statement. Obstet Gynecol Mar. 2020;135(3):e110–32. https://doi.org/10.1097/AOG.0000000000003719.
59. WHO recommendations for the prevention and management of tobacco use and second-hand smoke exposure in pregnancy. (2013) p. 104.
60. Higgins MF, Foley MC, Michael O'HC. Real increasing incidence of hysterectomy for placenta accreta following previous caesarean section. Eur J Obstet Gynecol Reprod Biol. 2013;171:54–6. https://doi.org/10.1016/j.ejogrb.2013.08.030.
61. Cheong YC, Bajekal N, Li TC. Peritoneal closure–to close or not to close. Hum Reprod. 2001;16:1548–52.
62. Palacios-Jaraquemada JM, D'Antonio F. Placenta Accreta Spectrum disorder: uterine dehiscence, not placental invasion. Obstet Gynecol. 2020;136(3):631. https://doi.org/10.1097/AOG.0000000000004071.
63. Sumigama S, Sugiyama C, Kotani T, Hayakawa H, Inoue A, Mano Y, Tsuda H, Furuhashi M, Yamamuro O, Kinoshita Y, Okamoto T, Nakamura H, Matsusawa K, Sakakibara K, Oguchi H, Kawai M, Shimoyama Y, Tamakoshi K, Kikkawa F. Uterine sutures at prior caesarean section and placenta accreta in subsequent pregnancy: a case-control study. BJOG. 2014;121(7):866–74. https://doi.org/10.1111/1471-0528.12717. discussion 875. Epub 2014 Mar 26
64. Di Spiezio SA, Saccone G, McCurdy R, Bujold E, Bifulco G, Berghella V. Risk of cesarean scar defect following single–versus double-layer uterine closure: systematic review and meta-analysis of randomized controlled trials. Ultrasound Obstet Gynecol. 2017;50:578–83.
65. Bamberg C, Dudenhausen JW, Bujak V, Rodekamp E, Brauer M, Hinkson L, Kalache K, Henrich W. A prospective randomized clinical trial of single vs. double layer closure of Hysterotomy at the time of cesarean delivery: the effect on uterine scar thickness. Ultraschall Med. 2018;39(3):343–51. https://doi.org/10.1055/s-0042-112223. Epub 2016 Sep 14
66. Kalem Z, Kaya AE, Bakırarar B, et al. An optimal uterine closure technique for better scar healing and avoiding isthmocele in CS: a randomized controlled study. J Investig Surg. 2019;9:1–9.
67. Antila-Långsjö RM, Mäenpää JU, Huhtala HS, Tomás EI, Staff SM. Cesarean scar defect: a prospective study on risk factors. Am J Obstet Gynecol. 2018;219(5):458.e1–8. https://doi.org/10.1016/j.ajog.2018.09.004.
68. SMFM Publication Committee. SMFM Consult Series #49; Russell Miller; Ilan E. Timor-Tritsch; Cynthia Gyamfi-Bannerman. (2020). Cesarean scar pregnancy. AJOG MFM.
69. Ishihara O, Araki R, Kuwahara A, Itakura A, Saito H, Adamson GD. Impact of frozen-thawed single blastocyst transfer on maternal and neonatal outcome: an analysis of 277,042 single-embryo transfer cycles from 2008 to 2010 in Japan. Fertil Steril. 2014;101(1):128–33.
70. Wikland M, Hardarson T, Hillensjo T, et al. Obstetric outcomes after transfer of vitrified blastocysts. Hum Reprod. 2010;25(7):1699–707.
71. Kaser DJ, Melamed A, Bormann CL, et al. Cryopreserved embryo transfer is an independent risk factor for placenta accreta. Fertil Steril. 2015;103(5):1176–1184.e2.
72. Silver RM. Placenta accreta syndrome. Portland, OR: CRC Press. Taylor & Francis Group; 2017. p. 5–6. Identifiers: LCCN 2016044635
73. Jauniaux E, Bhide A, Kennedy A, Woodward P, Hubinont C, Collins S. FIGO placenta Accreta diagnosis and management expert consensus panel. FIGO consensus guidelines on placenta accreta spectrum disorders: prenatal diagnosis and screening. Int J Gynaecol Obstet. 2018;140(3):274–80. https://doi.org/10.1002/ijgo.12408.
74. Shainker SA, Coleman B, Timor-Tritsch IE, Bhide A, Bromley B, Cahill AG, Gandhi M, Hecht JL, Johnson KM, Levine D, Mastrobattista J, Philips J, Platt LD, Shamshirsaz AA, Shipp TD, Silver RM, Simpson LL, Copel JA, Abuhamad A. Special report of the SMFM placenta Accreta

Spectrum ultrasound marker task force: consensus on definition of markers and approach to the ultrasound examination in pregnancies at risk for placenta accreta spectrum. Am J Obstet Gynecol. 2021;224(1):B2–B14. https://doi.org/10.1016/j.ajog.2020.09.001.
75. Zosmer N, Fuller J, Shaikh H, Johns J, Ross JA. Natural history of early first-trimester pregnancies implanted in cesarean scars. Ultrasound Obstet Gynecol. 2015;46:367–75.
76. D'Antonio F, Timor-Tritsch IE, Palacios-Jaraquemada J, et al. First trimester detection of abnormally invasive placenta in high-risk women: systematic review and meta-analysis. Ultrasound Obstet Gynecol. 2018;51:176–83. https://doi.org/10.1002/uog.18840.
77. Calì G, Timor-Trisch IE, Palacios-Jaraquemada J, et al. Changes in ultrasonography indicators of abnormally invasive placenta during pregnancy. Int J Gynaecol Obstet. 2018;140:319–25. https://doi.org/10.1002/ijgo.12413.
78. Timor-Tritsch IE, Monteagudo A, Cali G, Vintzileos A, Viscarello R, Al-Khan A, Zamudio S, Mayberry P, Cordoba MM, Dar P. Cesarean scar pregnancy is a precursor of morbidly adherent placenta. Ultrasound Obstet Gynecol. 2014;44(3):346–53. https://doi.org/10.1002/uog.13426. Epub 2014 Jul 31
79. Timor-Tritsch IE, Monteagudo A, Cali G, El Refaey H, Agten AK, Arslan AA. Easy sonographic differential diagnosis between intrauterine pregnancy and cesarean delivery scar pregnancy in the early first trimester. Am J Obstet Gynecol. 2016;215(2):225.e1–7. https://doi.org/10.1016/j.ajog.2016.02.028. Epub 2016 Feb 17
80. Timor-Tritsch IE, D'Antonio F, Calí G, Palacios-Jaraquemada J, Meyer J, Monteagudo A. Early first-trimester transvaginal ultrasound is indicated in pregnancy after previous cesarean delivery: should it be mandatory? Ultrasound Obstet Gynecol Aug. 2019;54(2):156–63. https://doi.org/10.1002/uog.20225. Epub 2019 Jul 10
81. Makukhina T. Early gestational ultrasound examination for placenta accreta spectrum disorder prediction. Ultrasound Obstet Gynecol. 2021;58(Suppl. 1):280–1. https://doi.org/10.1002/uog.24637.
82. Timor-Tritsch IE, Khatib N, Monteagudo A, Ramos J, Berg R, Kovács S. Cesarean scar pregnancies: experience of 60 cases. J Ultrasound Med. 2015;34(4):601–10. https://doi.org/10.7863/ultra.34.4.601.
83. Calì G, Timor-Trisch IE, Palacios-Jaraquemada J, et al. Outcome of cesarean scar pregnancy: A systematic review and meta-analysis. Ultrasound Obstet Gynecol. 2017;51:169. https://doi.org/10.1002/uog.17568. [Epub ahead of print].
84. Cali G, Forlani F, Timor-Tritsch IE, Palacios-Jaraquemada J, Minneci G, D'Antonio F. Natural history of cesarean scar pregnancy on prenatal ultrasound: the crossover sign. Ultrasound Obstet Gynecol. 2017;50(1):100–4. https://doi.org/10.1002/uog.16216. Epub 2017 Jun 7
85. El-Refaey H, El-Hibri F, Youakim N. Commentary 'all women with prior CS should have a 6- to 8-week scan to predict placenta accreta'. BJOG. 2014;140:171–82.
86. Linee guida Societ `a Italiana di Ecografia Ostetrica e Ginecologica e Metodologie Biofisiche. (2015) November. (SIEOG). https://www.sieog.it.
87. Desai N, Krantz D, Roman A, Fleischer A, Boulis S, Rochelson B. Elevated first trimester PAPP–a is associated with increased risk of placenta accreta. Prenat Diagn. 2014;34(2):159–62. https://doi.org/10.1002/pd.4277.
88. Thompson O, Otigbah C, Nnochiri A, et al. First trimester maternal serum biochemical markers of aneuploidy in pregnancies with abnormally invasive placentation. BJOG. 2015;122:1370–6.
89. Lyell DJ, Faucett AM, Baer RJ, et al. Maternal serum markers, characteristics and morbidly adherent placenta in women with previa. J Perinatol. 2015;35:570–4.
90. Penzhoyan GA, Makukhina TB. Significance of the routine first-trimester antenatal screening program for aneuploidy in the assessment of the risk of placenta accreta spectrum disorders. J Perinat Med. 2019;48(1):21–6. https://doi.org/10.1515/jpm-2019-0261.

Chapter 13
Setting Up a Referral Center for Placenta Accreta Spectrum

Sarah Tounsi, Karin A. Fox, Michael A. Belfort, and Ahmed A. Nassr

Introduction

The incidence of placenta accreta spectrum (PAS) continues to increase worldwide paralleling the increased rates of cesarean section [1] and other gynecologic and reproductive interventions. Given the magnitude of the problem, and the technical expertise and resources required to manage these patients safely, "centers of excellence" (CoE) have been established in many countries. While this is prudent, and is to be commended, the lack of a standardized definition of what constitutes a CoE and meaningful oversight complicates the issue. It thus behooves us to establish criteria for those institutions who claim the distinction of being a PAS referral center CoE and to be clear about what it takes to truly be a CoE as defined by outcomes and best practices, not just in name. By definition, a CoE is "a specialized program within healthcare institutions which supply exceptionally high concentrations of expertise and related resources centered on particular medical areas and delivered in a comprehensive, interdisciplinary fashion" [2].

In 2015, the American College of Obstetricians and Gynecologists (ACOG) and Society of Maternal Fetal Medicine (SMFM) developed a system for risk-appropriate maternal care facilities. This system is based on the expertise of the medical team and the region of operation. The aim was to reduce the overall maternal morbidity and mortality in the USA [3]. This is the basis of the levels of maternal care (MLOC) system which is now operational in many states. In the MLOC system, hospital designation is defined in a manner similar to the neonatal ICU designation system, whereby Level I centers offer the most basic level of care and Level IV centers offer comprehensive, complex, multidisciplinary care for the highest-risk patients. Both

S. Tounsi · K. A. Fox · M. A. Belfort · A. A. Nassr (✉)
Department of Obstetrics and Gynecology, Baylor College of Medicine and Texas Children's Hospital, Houston, TX, USA
e-mail: Ahmed.Nassr@bcm.edu

S. A. Shazly, A. A. Nassr (eds.), *Placenta Accreta Spectrum*,
https://doi.org/10.1007/978-3-031-10347-6_13

the ACOG and SMFM strongly recommend that patients who have PAS receive both medical and surgical care at a high-level center (MLOC III or higher) [4]. In 2021, the state of Texas has enacted a law (SB1164) requiring women with PAS to be referred to an MLOC III or IV facility for evaluation and management. Management in a facility with a designated program and multidisciplinary team has been shown to significantly improve maternal morbidity and mortality in PAS patients [4]. Specifically, women who deliver in such centers are at a reduced risk for needing a massive transfusion and for being subjected to re-operation when compared with delivery in a less specialized setting [5]. Despite published recommendations, as of 2013, only 25% of obstetricians polled by ACOG reported that they regularly referred patients with suspected PAS to a CoE [6]. We aim to describe the conditions and resources required to set up a PAS CoE and to highlight potential questions a referring provider and patient should ask of referral centers.

What Constitutes a PAS Center of Excellence?

Ideal management begins with early and accurate identification and diagnosis of PAS, preferably in the early antenatal period. This is accomplished mostly using ultrasound during the second trimester anatomy survey; however, cesarean scar implantation and signs of developing PAS may be seen in the first trimester. Magnetic resonance imaging (MRI) may be used (but is often not required) as an adjunctive imaging modality [7, 8]. Regardless of the imaging modality used, much of the diagnostic accuracy depends upon the experience of the examiner and quality of imaging obtained; therefore, expertise in obstetric imaging is crucial in order to ensure accurate, and timely, diagnosis, which significantly improve maternal outcome [9].

Adequate coordination of a multidisciplinary team comprised of personnel with the necessary expertise and skills is key for any PAS CoE. The "team of teams" should consist of, but not be limited to, specialists in maternal-fetal medicine (MFM), imaging (ultrasound and other forms of imaging), pelvic surgery (i.e., gynecologic oncology or urogynecology), obstetrical anesthesia, general surgery, vascular surgery, urology, interventional radiology, neonatology, and blood transfusion. Skilled nursing leadership, particularly those with experience in the management of postpartum hemorrhage and patients of high surgical acuity, should be involved [4, 10]. This broad range of expertise is highly recommended given the unpredictability of PAS during the course of pregnancy and the likelihood of need for complex surgery and the possible surgical complications that may arise at any given time.

While all of the members of every team may not be actively involved in every PAS case, it is essential that they be aware and ready to respond when such cases are planned and carried out. Since most CoE hospitals will be major obstetric referral centers, it is essential that the members of the PAS team be available on a 24/7 basis for these patients given the unpredictability of outside referrals and of the onset of labor or bleeding that may necessitate delivery ahead of schedule [9] (Fig. 13.1).

Concise and up-to-date guidelines should be available for all team members including those addressing preoperative, intraoperative, and postoperative care [9]. As far as is possible, all patients should be evaluated preoperatively in the PAS center ahead of time to ensure ample time for multidisciplinary team planning, patient counseling, and coordination of care. Many centers present their known cases at a multidisciplinary conference in order to discuss the planning, preparation, and timing of delivery. Any unique medical and social issues for the case are also reviewed [10].

The importance of an adequately staffed and supplied blood bank cannot be overemphasized. Sufficient blood products to allow an ongoing massive transfusion should be available 24/7. Whole blood packed red blood cells, fresh frozen plasma, cryoprecipitate, platelets, cell-saver technology, tranexamic acid, and lyophilized fibrinogen concentrate (Riastap®) should all be readily available [11–13].

PAS surgeries can be extremely complex and carry a high risk of maternal morbidity. Patients can rapidly become hemodynamically unstable and are at risk for rebleeding and reoperation. For this reason, postoperative recovery is often carried

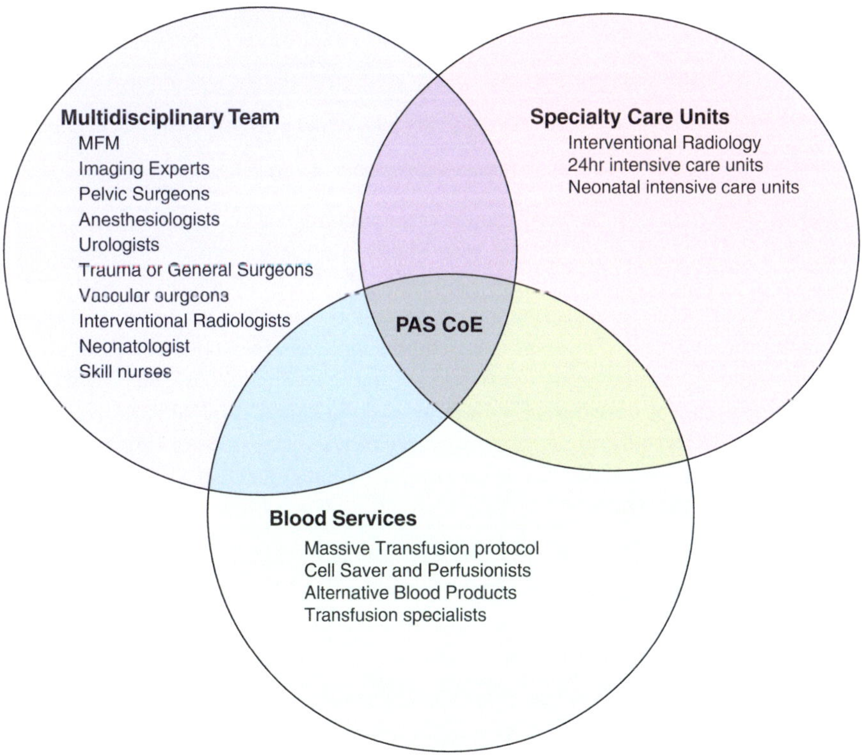

Fig. 13.1 Criteria for placenta accreta spectrum center of excellence

out in intensive care setting [10] where the one-to-one nursing-to-patient ratio and availability of sophisticated respiratory and cardiovascular support allow a rapid and comprehensive response to any emergency.

A Quick Overview

Every PAS center of excellence should have its own checklists for admission, surgical process, and postoperative recovery. The patient is typically admitted to the PAS CoE 5–7 days prior to surgery for controlled preparation. Once the patient is admitted, a standardized order set is used by the physician to ensure all necessary consults, blood testing, and blood bank preparations are made in a timely way. A paper checklist is completed by the patient's primary nurse and kept in the chart.

If the patient begins to bleed unexpectedly or go into labor, the team will be notified immediately and the on-call team can respond within 30 min. In our institution the MFM team will be notified first, and once the patient is evaluated, the other multidisciplinary teams involved are called in as required. The OR staff is always notified at the same time as the anesthesiology team, blood bank personnel, and neonatal ICU so that all of the teams are working contemporaneously toward the surgery [14].

Research

Progress in the field of PAS management is an ongoing endeavor, and it is important that PAS CoEs, regardless of their size, should be transparent in their outcomes (with quality improvement programs and committees and public disclosure of outcomes) and as much as possible engage in collaborative or individual institution research programs [14]. The level of research support varies between different centers and is highly dependent on the volume of patients seen at that CoE. For smaller centers, the ability to collaborate with larger similar centers and networks becomes important [14]. Given the increasing incidence of PAS (now around 1:500 deliveries in the USA), well-powered studies can now be contemplated if CoEs are open to collaborate with each other.

Conclusion

Patient safety is clearly the highest priority and responsibility for any prospective or established PAS CoE. Institutional and community support of a multidisciplinary team is a key, and crucial, component of any PAS CoE. Potential challenges include internal and external resistance from colleagues, referring doctors, and competing institutions, financial demands, and possible negative publicity around any unfortunate maternal outcomes [8]. However, it is important for the clinicians, administrators, and community to stay focused on the bigger clinical picture during the development of a CoE and on the goal which is to decrease maternal morbidity and mortality in patients with PAS and to provide the best possible medical and surgical care.

References

1. Organization WH. Caesarean section rates continue to rise, amid growing inequalities in access. Geneva: World Health Organization; 2021.
2. Elrod JK, Fortenberry JL. Centers of excellence in healthcare institutions: what they are and how to assemble them. BMC Health Serv Res. 2017;17(1):15–24.
3. Obstetricians ACo, Gynecologists. Obstetric care consensus no. 2: levels of maternal care. Obstet Gynecol. 2015;125(2):502–15.
4. Cahill AG, Beigi R, Heine RP, Silver RM, Wax JR, et al. Placenta accreta spectrum. Am J Obstet Gynecol. 2018;219(6):B2–B16.
5. Eller AG, Bennett MA, Sharshiner M, Masheter C, Soisson AP, Dodson M, et al. Maternal morbidity in cases of placenta accreta managed by a multidisciplinary care team compared with standard obstetric care. Obstet Gynecol. 2011;117(2):331–7.
6. Wright JD, Silver RM, Bonanno C, Gaddipati S, Lu Y-S, Simpson LL, et al. Practice patterns and knowledge of obstetricians and gynecologists regarding placenta accreta. J Matern Fetal Neonatal Med. 2013;26(16):1602–9.
7. Warshak CR, Ramos GA, Eskander R, Benirschke K, Saenz CC, Kelly TF, et al. Effect of predelivery diagnosis in 99 consecutive cases of placenta accreta. Obstet Gynecol. 2010;115(1):65–9.
8. Warshak CR, Eskander R, Hull AD, Scioscia AL, Mattrey RF, Benirschke K, et al. Accuracy of ultrasonography and magnetic resonance imaging in the diagnosis of placenta accreta. Obstet Gynecol. 2006;108(3):573–81.
9. Chandraharan E, Hartopp R, Thilaganathan B, Coutinho CM. How to set up a regional specialist referral service for placenta Accreta Spectrum (PAS) disorders? Best Pract Res Clin Obstet Gynaecol. 2021;72:92–101.
10. Silver RM, Fox KA, Barton JR, Abuhamad AZ, Simhan H, Huls CK, et al. Center of excellence for placenta accreta. Am J Obstet Gynecol. 2015;212(5):561–8.
11. Eller A, Porter T, Soisson P, Silver R. Optimal management strategies for placenta accreta. BJOG Int J Obstet Gynaecol. 2009;116(5):648–54.
12. Pri-Paz S, Fuchs KM, Gaddipati S, Lu Y-S, Wright JD, Devine PC. Comparison between emergent and elective delivery in women with placenta accreta. J Matern Fetal Neonatal Med. 2013;26(10):1007–11.
13. Shamshirsaz AA, Fox KA, Salmanian B, Diaz-Arrastia CR, Lee W, Baker BW, et al. Maternal morbidity in patients with morbidly adherent placenta treated with and without a standardized multidisciplinary approach. Am J Obstet Gynecol. 2015;212(2):218.e1-.e9.
14. Fox KA, Shamshirsaz AA, Belfort MA. Center of excellence for morbidly adherent placenta. Placenta Accreta Syndrome: CRC Press; 2017. p. 113–22.

Chapter 14
Management of PAS in Low-Resource Settings

Dema Adwan, Ahed Hamed, Mustafa Albokai, and Mhd Ali Alabdulrazak

Introduction

Placenta accreta spectrum (PAS) disorders are considered a potentially life-threatening complication of pregnancy that impacts maternal health globally [1]. PAS is associated with serious morbidities, primarily related to massive hemorrhage with associated organ damage, cesarean hysterectomy, and the need for critical care resources, with maternal morbidity in up to 60% of cases and mortality rate of up to 7% in affected patients [2–7]. The incidence of PAS has dramatically increased in the last 20 years [3]. The main standardized approach is hysterectomy and has remained so since the first reported cases [8, 9]. As PAS is a major problem for high-income countries, low-income countries face a critical situation in managing such cases of maximum seriousness. Having said that, to achieve safer outcomes in these poor settings, a variety of approaches emerged as a way to adapt to some crucial circumstances: the limited access to experienced surgeons, the lack of multidisciplinary teams (MDT) and insufficient infrastructure, and the absence of the intensive care recommended by the related guidelines [4]. This chapter aims to highlight some of the approaches used to manage PAS cases in low-income countries, such as Syria, as well as to evaluate the correspondence of these approaches to the current evidence-based guidelines.

D. Adwan (✉)
Department of Obstetrics & Gynecology, Damascus University, Damascus, Syria

University Hospital of Obstetrics and Gynecology, Damascus University, Damascus, Syria

A. Hamed
Department of Obstetrics & Gynecology, Damascus University, Damascus, Syria

Al Zahrawi Maternity Hospital, Damascus, Syria

M. Albokai · M. A. Alabdulrazak
Faculty of Medicine, Damascus University, Damascus, Syria

S. A. Shazly, A. A. Nassr (eds.), *Placenta Accreta Spectrum*, https://doi.org/10.1007/978-3-031-10347-6_14

Prenatal Diagnosis

Prenatal diagnosis of PAS is associated with a reduced risk of maternal complications such as peripartum hemorrhage, need for blood transfusions, and rate of hysterectomy, as it plays a crucial role in planning for the management of the condition [6, 9–15].

As outlined in a recent Obstetrics Care Consensus, obstetric ultrasonography is the primary screening modality for PAS [10, 16]. In addition, it is a relatively inexpensive and widely available imaging tool and therefore should be classified as the first line for the diagnosis of PAS [12]. The obstetric ultrasound continues to be the recommended first-choice procedure for diagnosing PAS not only in developed but also in the middle- and low-income countries; hence, this practice applies to our region [4, 10].

Markers of PAS can be detected by ultrasonography as early as the first trimester; however, in most women, the diagnosis is made in the second and third trimesters. Ideally, women with risk factors for PAS, such as placenta previa and previous cesarean delivery, should be assessed by obstetrician-gynecologists or other healthcare providers with enough expertise in diagnosing PAS by ultrasonography [10].

Although visualization of PAS findings on ultrasonography can be useful in diagnosis, none of the features (or combinations of features) associated with the PAS reliably predicts the depth of invasion or the type of placenta accreta spectrum [17]. This explains the role of other major tools used for the antenatal diagnosis of PAS, such as magnetic resonance imaging (MRI) that is recommended to complement ultrasound imaging in assessing the depth of invasion and lateral extension of myometrial invasion, especially in cases with posterior placentation or in women with ultrasound signs suggesting parametrial invasion [10, 11, 17–19].

It is uncertain whether MRI improves the diagnosis of PAS beyond that carried out with ultrasonography [17, 20]. Moreover, MRI is more expensive and less widely available, especially in low-income countries such as our region. Accordingly, MRI is not the preferred recommended modality for the initial evaluation of possible PAS because of the lack of proof of a clear value and the existence of downsides worthy of consideration [21].

Ultrasound Approach and Placenta Accreta Spectrum Markers

Starting with transabdominal imaging obtains an overview of the placental location and the regions of concern. Transvaginal ultrasonography (TVUS) is strongly recommended for assessing PAS. TVUS optimizes resolution and allows for a detailed assessment of the lower uterine segment, posterior bladder wall, and cervix [16]. As measuring cervical length in asymptomatic women with placenta previa can help in their management decision, a short cervical length measured on TVUS before 34 weeks with a partially full bladder is associated with increased risk of preterm delivery and massive hemorrhage at cesarean section [11]. Color Doppler should be utilized to determine vascularity and placental extension into the uterine wall and surrounding structures [16].

While assessing the placental location, placenta previa or a low-lying placenta should be searched for and detected antenatally as well [16].

We recommend that if a low-lying placenta or placenta previa is suspected during the routine scan, a follow-up ultrasound examination including a TVUS at 32 weeks of gestation should be made to diagnose persistent low-lying placenta and/or placenta previa cases. Besides, if proven at 32 weeks and the patient remained asymptomatic, we advocate another TVUS at around 36 weeks of gestation followed by a discussion about the best method of delivery.

Ultrasound image magnification should also be performed to enhance the visualization of target regions, for example, perpendicular orientation of the insonation angle and applying minimal transducer pressure when assessing the retroplacental region [16].

Given the disease continuum from cesarean scar pregnancy (CSP) to PAS and the fact that CSP markedly increases the risk of PAS, screening for PAS should begin early in the first trimester and continue throughout the pregnancy until practitioners conclude on the sonographic concerns for PAS [22–24]. Nonetheless, in our region, many CSP cases do not undergo early screening and present with complications later during pregnancy.

In Syria, markers outlined in the latest obstetric consensus are applied by obstetric-gynecologist experts in evaluating women with suspected PAS. Using these markers is of high significance especially in low-income countries as they improved the prenatal diagnosis of PAS, thus implementing the appropriate procedures available under low settings.

First-Trimester Evaluation

The prevalence and type of markers of PAS vary between the early first trimester of pregnancy (6–9 weeks of gestation) and the later first trimester of pregnancy (11–14 weeks of gestation) [22].

As mentioned earlier, when performing TVUS the maternal bladder should be partially filled enough to allow for a sonographic window, but without overfilling which can result in distortion of the uterovesical interface [16].

In patients with a previous cesarean delivery, implantation of a gestational sac in the lower uterine segment on ultrasound early in the first trimester is one of the most common markers for PAS in this period. Whence, a detailed evaluation of the uterus is necessary [25].

However, in the late first trimester, low implantation of the gestational sac is identified [22].

Anterior placentation at the first-trimester sonographic evaluation is more common in women with PAS at delivery [22, 26, 27]. Similar to findings in the second and third trimesters, the presence of multiple PAS markers in the first trimester increased the diagnostic accuracy [28–30].

Second- and Third-Trimester Evaluation

Previous papers traditionally described other markers in the second and third trimesters that were also detected in the late first trimester and are variably associated with PAS [28]. The definitions of the individual features are inconsistent but include the presence of placental lacunae, abnormal bladder interface, uterovesical hypervascularity, and loss of the retroplacental clear zone [22, 26, 27, 29].

Second- and third-trimester markers include placental lacunae (frequently described as classic ultrasound markers of PAS), abnormal uteroplacental interface, abnormal uterovesical interface, miscellaneous markers which include placental bulge, exophytic placental mass, and cervical vascular extension [16].

We assert that in order to strictly identify the risks and establish a better managing plan for each patient, such imaging findings should be discussed between the managing team and radiologists [1]. We also emphasize that although ultrasound is a significant modality in the diagnosis process, there are several limitations of its use in detecting PAS. Ultrasound is an imaging tool that depends on many factors, including the operator of the exam and his skills in performing the ultrasound [16]. This is mainly true in regions where there is a lack of ultrasonography expertise in identifying features of PAS [10].The detection rates will depend on the location of the placenta and maternal imaging conditions that impact the sonographic visualization of markers [16].

Despite optimizing a systematic approach to ultrasound examination for PAS markers, intrinsic limitations of ultrasound can lessen detection rates, including posterior placentation with limited sound penetration and resolution, elevated maternal BMI, and uterine leiomyomata [16].

Supposing the importance of ultrasound, the absence of ultrasound findings does not preclude a diagnosis of PAS. Thus, clinical risk factors remain as essential predictors of the placenta accreta spectrum by ultrasound findings [10].

Planning for Delivery

Where to Deliver?

Since the main risk associated with the delivery of patients diagnosed with PAS is massive hemorrhage and its related complications such as death, planning for delivery is crucial in minimizing morbidity and mortality rates [4, 11]. In addition, patients managed antenatally in a center of excellence (CoE) are less likely to require emergent surgery, large-volume blood transfusion, and reoperation within 7 days of delivery for bleeding complications compared with women managed by standard obstetric care without a specific protocol [31].

On that account, many protocols recommend that once the diagnosis of placenta accreta spectrum is made, a contingency plan for emergent delivery should be developed in partnership with the patient [4, 11, 12]. The delivery plan should include referring patients to a dedicated center so that delivery takes place in a specialist center with a multidisciplinary team (MDT), which will be discussed respectively, with expertise in complex pelvic surgeries and logistic support for immediate access to blood products, in addition to adult and neonatal intensive care units [3, 4, 11, 12].

We suggest informing the patients about the risks and solemnity of their condition and the consequences associated with deliveries in an unequipped center, along with discussing any possible choices.

If the patient's condition is stable and there are no episodes of bleeding, we can progress as an outpatient with a strict plan for delivery in a well-resourced setting. Yet, in a resource-poor setting with poor social circumstances (e.g., availability of emergency transport 24/7, patient education, and distance from the specialist center), the clinicians opt for hospitalization until delivery [32]. Despite the obstetrician's advice, many of them decline to accept in-house care due to multiple socioeconomic reasons and ultimately present with acute emergencies [33].

If patients are managed at home, they should be encouraged to ensure having safety precautions in place, including someone available to help them as necessary such as getting to the hospital [11, 34].

To sum up, all of the above are the best approaches to apply in our region especially when it comes to hospitalization decision that better be discussed upon their clinical status.

When to Deliver?

As for the timing of delivery, recent research is conflicting with varying recommendations, and the optimal timing of delivery for patients with PAS remains uncertain. Different protocols have been published ranging from 34–36 weeks to 36–38 weeks for non-emergent deliveries [15, 35, 36]. As pregnancy progresses in PAS patients, there is an increased risk for prepartum hemorrhage, and delivery beyond 36 weeks is not advisable because over half of these cases required emergency admission due to hemorrhage [9, 10]. Furthermore, non-emergent deliveries have better outcomes regarding maternal morbidity and blood loss, and preterm deliveries (34–35 weeks) showed a decrease in emergent deliveries reducing maternal mortality risk with no adverse effects on the fetus or the neonate [13–15].

In other situations, delivery must be at an earlier time as in cases of maternal morbidity development, membrane rupture, and persistent vaginal bleeding [10].

Thus, a PAS patient diagnosed early and managed electively at 34 to 36 weeks by an MDT in an adequately resourced center is required for optimal results, and planned preterm delivery is highly recommended in patients with episodes of contractions, prepartum hemorrhage, and PPROM [9]. We suggest this to be the best approach to be held in low-income countries considering the available recourses and the ability to manage emergent deliveries.

In Syria, we tend to extend the time of delivery beyond 36 weeks without complications as possible, as we do not have well-equipped neonatal intensive care units which would guarantee enough postoperative care for the baby if it was delivered at a sooner age.

Who Should Deliver?

Ideally as discussed before, patients with PAS should be managed by an MDT consisting of an obstetrician-gynecologist experienced with complex pelvic surgery in a specialist center, or preferably by the senior-most obstetrician and anesthetist in a minimum-equipped setting [3]. However, in low-setting centers when a trainee is attending the delivery in cases of emergency, the senior-most obstetrician and anesthetist should be alerted immediately and attend urgently toward avoiding profound maternal complications [11, 37].

MDT and Hospitalization

Appropriate management expertise is critical for an accreta center of excellence (CoE). Most authorities believe that outcomes regarding patients' safety are improved in a CoE with a well-established MDT [3, 9, 13, 15, 36, 38–40]. As a result, in such settings, the need for a second surgical operation and large volume blood transfusion is to a smaller extent, and patients are less likely to experience morbidity than those receiving obstetric care in traditional unequipped settings [13]. Significantly, more studies reported lower maternal mortality rates in cases of obstetric hemorrhage and better outcomes of emergency deliveries when performed in centers of excellence with MDTs that fit the criteria of the current evidence-based guidelines [15, 39].

As shown earlier, one of the fundamental factors to success in a PAS Center of Excellence is to have a multidisciplinary team of coordinated providers with enough expertise in managing PAS cases [16].

This is proven true, especially in low-income settings; to optimize the available resources and maternal health outcomes, the MDT approach is of utmost importance as resources and technical abilities are limited in such settings [4, 13, 15]. The optimal scenario is achieved when adopting this approach in the settings of elective operations, in an environment that is specifically designed for PAS management [3].

Consequently, for low-income countries, this applies as follows: women with a diagnosis of PAS should be referred to a regional center dedicated to the interdisciplinary management of the condition, where resources are concentrated and experts of multiple specialties assemble as an MDT while emphasizing that all cases of PAS (diagnosed prenatally or intraoperatively) should be treated in such center, for the experiences to accumulate and further improve the MDT ability [4].

Under concordant recommendations, an MDT should include the following: experts in imaging for diagnosis, experts in complex surgery (gynecologic oncology, pelvic surgeon, urogynecologist) and additional specialists for surgical complications (vascular surgeon, urologist), adult and neonatal intensive care units with the respective specialists, interventional radiologists, and a blood bank with massive transfusion protocols [3, 4, 9, 41]. In circumstances like ours, a gynecologist and a urologist are the only ones available most of the time, with access to vascular surgery specialists occasionally.

As for the timing of hospitalization, two different situations are recognized in Syria: elective and emergent cases.

I. In elective cases, hospital admission should be a few days before the scheduled timing of delivery, to evaluate the patient's hemodynamics and ability to undergo the operation (i.e., monitor Hb levels and perform blood transfusion if needed, renotify critical care units and blood bank, and get the MDT ready with fully equipped operation room). This applies to outpatient and inpatient elective surgeries, and then, hospitalization happens at age of 36 weeks of gestation. For outpatients specifically, patients should be aware and pay attention to any complication that may happen as they should report immediately to any hospital; this includes vaginal bleeding, membrane rupture, prepartum hemorrhage, and PPROM. Henceforth, an emergency hospitalization may be indicated.
II. In case of bleeding, the patient is to be hospitalized immediately and should remain so until the timing of delivery.

In preparation for delivery, the administration of corticosteroids is essential for fetal lung maturation [9]. Corticosteroids should be administered to all women with PAS as preterm delivery is very likely. Preferably, the administration should be at 34–36 weeks of gestation as a single-course therapy, and even earlier for patients who are at particular risk of preterm delivery [11, 41–43].

In our situation, it's performed earlier than week 34 of gestational age, and this is highly important in poor settings as there could be a lack of beds in neonatal care units.

On the other hand, in patients with symptomatic PAS, facilitation of corticosteroids administration could be considered, by performing tocolysis for 48 h as recommended in evidence-based guidelines, which is also applied in low-income countries. It is noteworthy to mention that tocolysis is indicated only in symptomatic PAS, not in other situations [44].

Due to the risk of prepartum hemorrhage in cases of PAS, hemoglobin levels should be monitored, especially since anemia is of high prevalence in pregnancy (as high as 38%), mostly caused by iron deficiency [9]. If iron deficiency is confirmed (hemoglobin level is less than 110 g/L before 28 weeks of gestation, or less than 105 g/L after 28 weeks of gestation), it should be corrected via oral supplements, intravenous injection, or erythropoiesis stimulation if indicated [4, 9–11, 45]. Unfortunately, in low-income countries, the recommendations regarding the correction of hemoglobin levels during pregnancy are not always put into consideration, due to many reasons: insufficient prenatal visits, socioeconomic status of the patient, and lacking awareness of the seriousness of the case.

In addition, preoperative measures must be taken, to properly manage complications if persistent hemorrhage occurred, and a blood bank should be notified in advance. Ideally, a blood bank should be able to perform massive transfusion protocols; prothrombin complex concentrate; coagulation factors VII, VIII, and IX; and prior cell salvage [4]. In poor settings, this criterion may not fit and only exists in a few centers. Thus, prior notification to said center and coordinated transport of the patient are essential while using volume expanders until the patient can receive a better level of care. Such procedures, tools, and facilities do not all exist in Syria.

The risk of venous thromboembolism development should also be estimated after hospitalization and balanced with the risk of hemorrhage from the low-lying placenta or placenta previa [11]. This is important due to the patient's bed rest and lack of movement and the possibility of massive bleeding, which all together increases the risk of venous thromboembolism. As a result, it is advised to use compression stockings to help minimize the risk [46, 47].

Another pivotal aspect is the availability of neonatal care units and neonatologists capable of providing round-the-clock services, managing any delivery whether planned or unexpected, and monitoring the neonate postoperatively due to some possible complications (related to PAS or not) occurring after delivery [15]. To the extent of enhancing neonatal health outcomes in poor settings, hospitalization of PAS patients should ideally be scheduled in terms of informing the neonatologists about its indication and gestational age with emphasis on early lung maturation of the fetus. This is crucial due to the probability of lacking neonatal care resources in such settings [4, 48].

Overall, to achieve high-quality care that is in alignment with guidelines recommendations in such poor settings, multiple elements should be guaranteed: the pre-operative planning should include a multidisciplinary involvement with an emphasis on consultant anesthesiologist and obstetrician role in planning and direct supervision over the operation, with free access to a fully operational blood bank with the available blood products and availability of level 2 critical care beds [11, 49].

Surgical Management

Many debates have been held about the optimal surgical approach for antenatally suspected placenta accreta spectrum, as there yet to be no RCTs comparing different surgical techniques. Note that a high rate of maternal morbidity continues to exist irrespective of the approach to be conservative or radical, though an experienced staff in a specialized facility can significantly reduce possible risks [3, 13, 15, 36, 40, 57].

It is worth mentioning the factors affecting the decision of the proper surgical approach: the position of the placenta, depth of invasion, the parametrial extension of the PAS as evaluated by ultrasound and/or MRI before delivery, visual assessment of the uterus at the time of surgery, and the presenting clinical symptoms like bleeding [11, 34, 58].

Referring to the previous point about early diagnosis and its associated better outcomes, the patient and her partner must be fully briefed and counseled about any treatment options and their potential effects [16]. This includes gaining consent for cesarean hysterectomy and informing the patient about the risk of sepsis and delayed hemorrhage that can occur when the uterus is conserved with the placenta left in situ, also about the possibility of proceeding from conservative to radical methods if needed [11].

Urologic Injury

Urologic injury is a potential complication when it comes to PAS surgical management, especially associated with standard hysterectomy. Thus, modification of the surgical techniques is essential to minimize the risk of such injuries [59].

One of the followed procedures is the preoperative placement of ureteric stents. Research has shown that it can reduce the risk of urologic injury from 33% to 6%, but it has also shown that its use is attributed to the surgeon's preference and is not always performed [4, 60]. Accordingly, ureteric stents are not commonly used in Syria due to lack of availability.

Cystoscopic assessment is another procedure that influences the urologic tract injury. It provides evidence of placental invasion of the bladder, thus alarming the surgeon to be aware of the situation and providing extra caution while dissecting the bladder [9, 60, 61]. Hence, in a situation like ours, it is recommended to perform cystoscopy in case of suspected invasion of the bladder by the placenta percreta, if indicated by the prenatal imaging or the patient presents with hematuria.

Type of Incisions for Access

Mostly, a midline incision is recommended for PAS disorders diagnosed prenatally or at the time of cesarean delivery [9, 15, 36, 59, 62, 63].

However, in Syria, Pfannenstiel's incision is the most used surgical incision. On the other hand, the para-midline incision is rarely used, even by urological surgeons if they were summoned during the surgical procedure as it could be a conservative approach and for consideration of the psychological aspect of the patient as there is a possibility that she would undergo a hysterectomy which in turn could affect her psychological condition.

Blood Conservation Techniques

Various procedures and techniques can reduce the risk of blood loss and conserve blood volume either preoperatively or intraoperatively [9].

Tranexamic acid, a hemostatic antifibrinolytic agent, is wildly used to control hemorrhage and proved to significantly reduce hemorrhage-associated mortality. Unfortunately, it is not used in settings like ours [9, 64–66].

Balloon occlusion catheters are also used to control blood loss by inflating a balloon catheter in major arteries with interventional radiology guidance. As opposed, evidence of its efficacy is still lacking, and its use is controversial due to potential risks [11, 67]. For that reason, it is not recommended for routine use yet including in our country due to the unavailability of interventional radiology facilities.

Another procedure is internal iliac artery ligation, of which the advantages are comparable to those of balloon occlusion catheter, but with an additional advantage of the possibility of application in poor-resource settings as it does not require specialized facilities. There is still insufficient evidence about which of the prior two procedures has better outcomes [1]. It is worth mentioning that artery ligation is used intraoperatively in our case when indicated.

On the other hand, some centers adopted the cell salvage technique as a measure to reduce the need for blood product transfusion despite being relatively expensive [9, 68–70]. As follows, its cost-benefit ratio is not favorable in our settings.

More importantly, no attempt to remove the placenta should be taken if PAS was suspected or diagnosed intraoperatively, as removal in cases of PAS is known to trigger massive uncontrolled hemorrhage. This is particularly essential in situations where access to blood transfusion is limited [6, 9, 13, 40].

In a hysterectomy procedure for treating PAS, manual separation of the placenta should be avoided as well as uterotonic agents, that is, leaving the placenta in situ is associated with lower blood loss. In specific cases where the placenta spontaneously separates to some extent with limited invasion in depth and width, conservative approaches could be employed and the choice of such approaches is dependent on the specifics of the new situation; therefore, uterotonic agents could be administered if enough separation occurred, or in cases of total spontaneous placental separation, thus ruling out PAS as a diagnosis [9, 59].

Surgical Methods

The method of choice in managing PAS is dependent on multiple factors, namely, the patient's wish for future fertility, preoperative and intraoperative findings, and if the situation allows for conservative treatment or not [71]. If the conservative management is not an option or the patient did not opt for it, the method of choice is en bloc resection of the uterus with the placenta left in situ. While there are various approaches for conservative treatment, the risk for morbidity and safety of such procedures is debatable [4, 10, 71].

After placing the patient in a lithotomy position for proper evaluation of intraoperative bleeding and placing of a urinary catheter, infusion of the bladder with 200 cc normal saline is advised, ideally with methylene blue dye. This procedure should be either applied in radical or conservative methods and can be re-applied multiple times during the operation.

It should be noted that the following steps are mutual in both conservative and radical approaches, and each of them will be detailed thoroughly.

- First, administration of anesthesia is initiated, and the abdominal incision is made.
- Once accessed to the abdominal cavity, observation and inspection of the pelvis is essential to visually assess the depth of placental invasion and recognize any adhesions caused by prior surgeries.
- Afterward, sharp bladder dissection is achieved before uterine incision toward the lower parts of the bladder while holding the posterior bladder wall with Babcock forceps [67]. This is an essential step and should be done carefully until

the cervix is reached. Bladder dissection before delivery is a key feature to reduce bladder injury, as it allows the identification of tissues properly and detection of the vescico-uterine plane before hemorrhage happens [9, 72].

- Major feeding vessels are to be secured and the abundant neovascularization should be stabilized, whether on the uterus or the bladder using bipolar electrocautery.
- The last two steps are essential in minimizing urologic injury by avoiding intra-operative bleeding that hampers visibility and requires urgent dissection of the bladder, which is already covered by a pool of blood, thus making it more difficult to get the vesico-uterine plane. As a result, neovascularization obstructs bladder dissection by causing major bleeding, especially in cases of percreta [9].
- In those cases of percreta where there is an extensive bulging of the thinned-out uterus into the posterior bladder wall, adopting a lateral approach in the dissection of the bladder could be the manner of choice; entrance between the two layers of the broad ligament after detaching the round ligament may allow stepwise devascularization of the uterus and may aid later in hysterectomy [9, 73].
- In cases of placenta percreta with bladder involvement, it is recommended to perform a cystotomy to identify the villous tissue and remove the involved segment of the bladder. The incision should be performed until it reaches ureters' opening to allow adequate dissection of the posterior segment of the bladder [9, 15, 59].
- After that, a hysterotomy incision is performed, ideally in the upper segment of the uterus to avoid the placental site. Some may proceed with exteriorization of the uterus outside the abdominal cavity through the abdominal incision, to gain better control and manipulation over the uterus and is helpful by causing tension over the arteries of the uterus and ovaries, thus reducing blood supply to the placenta [9, 74]. However, we tend to exteriorize the uterus immediately after the baby is born then close it with hemostatic sutures.
- At the delivery, the umbilical cord is cut, tied, and placed in the uterus while the baby is handed over to the neonatal team. Precautions should be considered to not disturb the placental bed. If the placenta is transected accidentally, immediately clamp the umbilical cord to stop fetal blood loss [11, 75].

If the diagnosis is set to be placenta percreta and was seen with the naked eye in the laparotomy, then we never wait for the placenta to be separated; we proceed with closing the uterine incision completely after leaving the placenta and execute emergent hysterectomy.

However, if the case was placenta increta and confirmed during surgery, it is possible not to wait for placental detachment and proceed immediately with hysterectomy, noting that there is a possibility that a part of the placenta could be separated during surgery leaving the other part inserted within the myometrium, hence treated with a conservative approach that will be mentioned later.

However, in the case of accreta, it is necessary to wait for 15 min maximum while holding the edges of the uterus; if the placenta completely separates spontaneously, then the diagnosis of PAS is excluded, but in case of partial separation, conservative management is the mean of choice with attention made to the necessity of hemostasis.

Conservative Techniques

Many techniques were described in the literature to control hemorrhage including uterine and endo-uterine compressive sutures. B-Lynch technique, described in 1997, is still the best-known suture technique [77]. Interestingly, a new method came out combining B-Lynch and the intrauterine balloon technique, which proved its success in preventing PPH in placenta previa [78].

- *Methotrexate (Mtx)*, a folate antagonist, was first described by Arul Kumaran et al. as an adjuvant therapy for the conservative management of placenta accreta. There has been a controversial conflict about its value actions with some arguing that it induces placental necrosis and promotes more rapid regression of the placenta and others specifying its action only on rapidly dividing cells, conflicting with the fact that trophoblastic proliferation does not occur after delivery and therefore finalizing that methotrexate is of no value.

  In addition, there has been a lack of randomized trials regarding its optimum dosing, frequency, or route of administration [76].

  In our settings, its use is limited to the presence of small focal placental remnants without severe bleeding. However, it is rarely used as it requires a prolonged hospitalization for the patient (3–4 months) for continuous monitoring of bleeding, and that is not acceptable in our society aside from being refused by the patient due to multiple socioeconomic reasons.
- *Triple P procedure* is also a conservative modified surgical technique, described in 2010 and applied when the placenta appears to be focal, that there is a portion of the placenta separates gradually while the other portion is engraved in the myometrium [32]. With knowing that focal adhesion is susceptive to wedge resection with complete removal of the placenta and repair of the uterus, considerations to this case may be given to the extension of the classical uterine incision, initiating the resecting of the placenta and implantation site [1]. *Triple P* procedure involves three steps, followed by a second step using interventional radiology before patient transfer to the obstetric theater [1]:

  1. Preoperative localization of the placenta and delivering fetus by incision above the upper border of the placenta
  2. Pelvic devascularization by inflating balloon catheter in both internal iliac arteries
  3. Placental non-separation with myometrial excision and uterine wall reconstruction

     Due to the lack of interventional radiology in our region, this procedure cannot be applied.
- *Tamponade techniques* use the cervix as a natural tamponade in controlling postpartum hemorrhage caused by placenta previa and placenta accreta [79–82]. This technique is not fairly used in our country, except for some surgeons.
- *Expectant management* is defined as leaving the placenta in situ, waiting for its complete spontaneous resorption, then followed by one of the multiple procedures, inclusive of administration of methotrexate, embolization of the internal iliac or uterine arteries, or other described procedures [11]. This is usually

inquired after an elective caesarian section encountered by an undiagnosed placenta accreta in an unequipped center for PAS emergencies.

- In Syria, whenever we come across the previous scenario, we close the hysterotomy incision immediately after delivering the baby, leaving the placenta in situ without any intervention, and then transfer the patient to a qualified multidisciplinary center to take the correspondent actions.
- In line with the procedure held in Syria in case of partial insertion of the placenta into the myometrium is the following detailed explanation:

1. Tie a Nylon fiber with a Vicryl one.
2. Make three knots and make sure of their stability.
3. Insert the needle of the Nylon fiber from the anterior wall of the uterine into the posterior wall at the level of the lower segment (site of accreta).
4. Pull the Nylon fiber with the Vicryl.
5. Insert the needle of the Nylon fiber from the posterior wall of the uterine into the anterior wall and pull the knot with the Vicryl fiber gently.
6. Ask the assistant surgeon to make sure of the permeability through the lower segment and not to be completely closed, in anticipation of hematoma formation over the suture.
7. Make sure that the knot is pulled enough.

- This procedure is considered as one of the compression suture types applied to the lower segment. As soon as it is completed, we should ensure that the walls of the uterus are tightened into each other at the level of the lower segment with the cervix left open for any amount of blood to drain, preventing the formation of a hematoma as described earlier.
- Unfortunately, if any bleeding is detected at the site of sutures, we should initiate with uterine artery ligation, and if bleeding continues, ligation of the anterior branches of internal iliac arteries would be the safest solution in hand, while uterine hysterectomy stands as the last definite option for a nonstop bleed
- In addition, due to the unavailability of Bakri balloon in our settings, we usually end this given procedure by placing a surgical mesh at the site of suturing before tying the knots (to avoid interfering within the mesh) and then extracting the mesh from the vagina to be withdrawn after 24 h on condition of no active bleeding in place.
- Concluding with, this procedure is best described as a modified and a similar conservative manner to what has been published in literature so far.

Radical Management

For many years, radical hysterectomy at the time of cesarean section has been the primary treatment of placenta accreta spectrum in case of postpartum hemorrhage, reducing the risk of its associated complications including injuries to adjacent pelvic organs, massive blood transfusions, disseminated intravascular coagulopathy, and high mortality rates [11].

On the contrary, recent research found that emergent hysterectomy is associated with maternal morbidity in 56% of cases and with a mortality rate of 3% [11].

Morbidities linked to hysterectomy differ from loss of fertility to complications including injury to the gastrointestinal or urinary tracts, infection, as well as massive obstetrical hemorrhage and its consequences [11].

Among types of hysterectomy, total hysterectomy is the preferred method for emergent peripartum hemorrhage as reported in a survey of SMFM specialists regarding their management of PAS disorders, with 55% of specialists performed total hysterectomy while 45% of subtotal procedure proponents [83].

Supporters of subtotal hysterectomy report decreased blood loss, blood transfusions, perioperative complications, and shorter operating times [60].

However, in cases of PAS disorders with deep invasion up to the serosa and thepresence of cervical involvement, subtotal hysterectomy may not be as effective. In addition, subtotal hysterectomy has not been shown to protect against urinary tract injury compared with total hysterectomy in surgeries for PAS, except for an increased likelihood of developing cervical adenocarcinoma over time [60]. Consequently, we suggest selecting a total hysterectomy approach in our region.

Steps of Classical Hysterectomy

If a hysterectomy has been decided at a cesarean section:

1. Start with closing the uterine incision with the placenta preserved inside.
2. After holding the round ligaments, cut and ligate on both sides, each separately, consecutively.
3. Dissect the anterior layer of the broad ligament and then open a window from which ligation of the adnexa is possible. Concerning recent studies, removing the adnexa diminishes subsequent development of adnexal carcinomas, if left without excision [60].
4. Begin with the infundibulopelvic ligament (suspensory ligament of the ovary), cut and ligate in both sides, each separately, consecutively, performing a free knot first, and then a trans-fixation to the cut edges.
5. Before clamping the uterine artery, in the absence of bleeding, it is better to detect the ureters directly. If an ectasis in the ureter is visualized, a urologist is called to probe it. Opening the retroperitoneal space and visualizing the ureters can be helpful and preventive from inadvertent damage to the ureters [9].
6. Clamp the uterine arteries on both sides at a time before cutting, to avoid recurrent bleeding.
7. Resort to ligation of the anterior branches of the internal iliac arteries only in case of major bleeding.
8. For cervical removal, a wedge-shaped section from each side is performed, and then the stumps are cut and tied.
9. Finally, the vaginal vault is suspended on the cardinal ligament with knots or locked sutures depending on the presence of bleeding

Toward ending the hysterectomy, more instructions should not be dispensed with:

1. Uttermost hemostasis should be achieved, by checking all the stumps that it is possible to apply a gelfoam sponge on any blood-oozing surfaces or the posterior surface of the bladder, or a tampon or two where it is pulled out from a separate wound in the abdomen and then removed after 24 h or more.
2. If the posterior wall of the bladder is damaged, it should be repaired with continuous unlocked sutures within the mucosa, whereas it is useful to repeat the injection of normal saline (preferably with methylene blue dye) within the bladder to ensure that the entire surface is intact.
3. Drainage placement is advised in most Cases

In cases of noticeable and ongoing hemorrhage, pharmacological measures are attempted and then surgical techniques for hemostasis are tried, respectively. Ligation of the round ligament as the first step of hysterectomy allows visualizing of the para-rectal and para-vesical spaces with access to the major pelvic vessels and the ureters. Then, the anterior branches of the internal iliac arteries should be ligated. Significantly, caution is advised at the time of iliac artery ligation, especially in poor settings, as the ureter is located anteriorly and the internal iliac vein posterolaterally; as a result, inexperienced operators should not attempt the procedure unsupervised. Once the ligation procedure is over, ovarian ligaments should be secured and transected.

Intraoperative Considerations According to Recent Guidelines [1]

- Pneumatic compression stockings may be considered if there is a predisposition for coagulation [84].
- IV antibiotics are to be given at skin incision [85].
- The upper anterior edge of the placenta should be located using ultrasonography, to guide the skin incision required for adequate uterus exposure [86].
- Identification of the anterior or posterior cervicovaginal margins is achieved by placement of an instrument in the vaginal fornices before excision of the uterus, such as the Breisky retractor [9].
- Inspection of the ureteric orifices is achieved by repeat cystoscopy following vault closure and before the closure of the abdomen [61].

We strongly suggest our practitioners stick to the previous considerations whenever available.

Planned Hysterectomy

Planned delayed hysterectomy is an alternative approach used in cases of severe invasion of the placenta (placenta percreta which makes immediate surgery difficult) and is usually performed after 3–12 weeks of the delivery [11]. Despite having positive effects such as decreased vascularity and absorption of the placenta, which in turn facilitates the second surgery, risks associated with it are mainly coagulopathy, hemorrhage, and sepsis [36].

While sometimes ligation of internal iliac arteries or embolization of uterine arteries could also cause complications, the patient's strict compliance with the doctor is required [9, 36, 87–89].

Generally, planned delayed hysterectomy is far from being approved or practiced in Syria.

Unexpected Placenta Accreta or Intraoperative Diagnosis

As outlined previously, antenatal consultation, early diagnosis, and planned delivery proved their role in improving pregnancy outcomes in patients with a suspected morbidly adherent placenta [6, 14, 41, 90].

Oppositely, PAS is occasionally discovered unintentionally during delivery, either before or after the baby is delivered, and attempts of placental removal are performed [10]. In this case, morbidity and mortality rates depend primarily on the immediate management made by the medical staff.

In similar situations, it is critical to check for active bleeding; assess the extent and location of placental invasion, which can range from a completely visible placenta upon entry into the abdomen to at or beyond the lower uterine segment with extension into the bladder or pelvic sidewalls; and consider the resources available [3].

The most crucial resources that should be available at the site of operation are professional surgeons as a part of a multidisciplinary team, as described earlier, and proper equipment [3].

Wherefore two cases could be faced, the patient is actively bleeding, or the patient is hemodynamically stable, yet there are no resources accessible in both scenarios.

While in the bleeding case it is essential to apply local pressure to the bleeding sites in the first place (except those where placental tissue is at risk), prepare for hysterotomy to deliver the baby followed by the appropriate management of choice whether radical or conservative after closing the hysterotomy incision and transferring the patient to the dedicated center.

Meanwhile, a pre-fascial closure intraoperative photograph could be delivered with the patient. This will improve the receiving facility's preoperative preparation. In addition, if the percreta is freshly detected and conservative management is being considered, intraoperative ultrasonography involving a probe enclosed in a sterile sleeve can be used to determine the placental position. This will help in determining the best hysterotomy site (fundal or even posterior uterine) to avoid disrupting the placenta's attachment to the uterine wall [3].

In Syria, unfortunately, some obstetricians may carry on with such operations despite a lack of resources and in a facility that is not well-equipped. For safety considerations, especially in low-setting circumstances, we recommend transferring the patient to a dedicated center with complete readiness without putting the lives of the mother and her baby under any possible risk.

Altogether, we also urge that all delivery centers consider the risk of PAS during delivery especially elective cesarean sections and that facilities should have immediate plans in place to deal with emergent situations as explained above.

Postoperative Care

After a complicated delivery, patients are transferred immediately to the intensive care unit to be carefully managed [11]. Their residency in ICU will be for around 24 h without any complications.

Strict instructions are given to the staff for monitoring the patient as there is a persistent risk for coagulopathy, anemia, thromboembolism, and renal, cardiac, and organ dysfunction [4].

Accordingly, many considerations were described for this critical period [4]:

1. Continuous monitoring and registering of patient's vital signs (body temperature, pulse rate, respiration rate, and blood pressure) as first signs to alter in case of bleeding which can be internal and not visualized.
2. Monitoring of urine output through a urinary catheter which is left in situ for 10 days (at least 1 week). This determines the amount of fluid to be compensated daily.
3. Regular tests that include daily CBC: hemoglobin level to evaluate the need for blood transfusion, platelet count for thrombotic condition, and WBC count as an indicator of possible infection, in addition to a complete profile of the liver and kidney functional status.
4. Intravenous prophylactic antibiotic coverage for 36–48 h and then converted orally.
5. Administration of anticoagulants to prevent deep vein thrombosis after 12 h.
6. Pain killers are also indicated

Proceeding 24 h of vital stability is the main factor that aids in determining the possibility of transferring the patient into the ward.

In conclusion, as previously demonstrated, we would like to emphasize the appropriate and effective strategies urgently needed for the identification and management of PAS disorders, given the high incidence and the clinical significance of PAS conditions, hence committing to the recommendations, which have been summarized throughout different sections, the collaboration of regional centers by conducting related research that will provide accurate data to boost the quality of healthcare provided, and putting in mind that our priority is the safety of the patient and her infant, even in low circumstances that do not compare with those in other developed countries.

Anesthetic Management

The decision of what type of anesthesia should be a result of integrated planning between the anesthesiologist and the MDT, to balance the risks and benefits of each type to fit the PAS case by its risk factors.

Multiple factors are usually taken into consideration, most notably the hemodynamic stability, risk of hemorrhage, potential intraoperative complications, and the patient's comorbidities.

Generally, recent guidelines reported that regional anesthesia reduces hemorrhage-related morbidities regarding blood loss and transfusion requirements and improves neonatal outcomes especially respiratory outcomes and Apgar score [4, 9]. But due to the risk of massive hemorrhage, general anesthesia should also be considered in some situations, especially in cases of high PAS suspicion [4, 9, 50–52].

Also, intraoperative conversion from regional to general anesthesia is probable if PAS is diagnosed intraoperatively, especially in cases of epidural anesthesia that causes sympathetic block leading to hemodynamic instability and increased risk for hemorrhage [3, 9]. As shown in recent papers, one size does not fit it all, as the choice is case-specific and is ultimately dependent on the anesthesiologist's assessment [53–56].

In summary, we point up some recommendations regardless of the anesthetic type used: establishing multiple venous access points (preferably large diameter veins for crystalloids and blood products), hemodynamic monitoring with an arterial line, and monitoring of central venous pressure, with the capacity to treat hypothermia [3, 4].

Conservative Management

Conservative management appeared to be a successful alternative to radical approaches and an option for women who desire to preserve their fertility [11].

Recently, there has been a shift away from the traditional cesarean hysterectomy (also known as the extirpative approach) toward more conservative approaches such as uterine conservation, which is defined as leaving the placenta in situ partially or totally with no attempt to remove it, followed by medical management in some cases including adjuvant treatment of methotrexate, uterine artery embolization, internal iliac artery ligation/embolization, dilatation and curettage (or hysteroscopic loop resection), or simply awaiting spontaneous resorption of the placenta [4, 76].

Leaving the placenta in situ reduces the risk of hemorrhage that can occur at the time of hysterectomy because of rich vascular plexus in the lower uterine segment; however, it is unrecommended if the patient presents with major bleeding as it is unlikely to be therapeutic and risks will delay conclusive treatment, thus increasing morbidity [76].

Conservative management comes as an option only in well-equipped centers as it requires enough preparations and requirements from facilities for embolization, blood bank, and a highly expert team of surgeons as there is a potential for initiating radical procedures in case of a failure while proceeding. Moreover, the capability of establishing a firm follow-up plan to encounter any complication is of utmost importance [76].

All guidelines emphasized close follow-up when managing conservatively, for the possibility of the development of any complications that may arise weeks or months after delivery [11].

On the flip side, there is continuous potential morbidity associated with conservative management including sepsis (involving septic shock), peritonitis, uterine necrosis, fistula, injury to the adjacent organs, acute pulmonary edema, acute renal failure, deep vein thrombophlebitis, pulmonary embolism, and death. Therefore, we note that women who choose this type of management, if clinically possible, should be aware of all the potential risks [76].

Fever is the most reported complication, which usually presents after endometritis or florid sepsis. In the absence of an infectious cause, fever could be an inflammatory reaction to tissue necrosis. The use of preventive broad-spectrum antibiotic treatment in the immediate postpartum period can reduce infectious morbidity [76].

References

1. Hobson SR, Kingdom JC, Murji A, Windrim RC, Carvalho JCA, Singh SS, et al. No. 383-screening, Diagnosis, and Management of Placenta Accreta Spectrum Disorders. J Obstet Gynaecol Can. 2019;41(7):1035–49.
2. Creanga AA, Bateman BT, Butwick AJ, Raleigh L, Maeda A, Kuklina E, et al. Morbidity associated with cesarean delivery in the United States: is placenta accreta an increasingly important contributor? Am J Obstet Gynecol. 2015;213(3):384 e1–11.
3. Silver RM, Fox KA, Barton JR, Abuhamad AZ, Simhan H, Huls CK, et al. Center of excellence for placenta accreta. Am J Obstet Gynecol. 2015;212(5):561–8.
4. Escobar MF, Gallego JC, Nasner D, Gunawardana K. Management of abnormal invasive placenta in a low- and medium-resource setting. Best Pract Res Clin Obstet Gynaecol. 2021;72:117–28.
5. Sumigama S, Itakura A, Ota T, Okada M, Kotani T, Hayakawa H, et al. Placenta previa increta/percreta in Japan: a retrospective study of ultrasound findings, management and clinical course. J Obstet Gynaecol Res. 2007;33(5):606–11.
6. Eller AG, Porter TF, Soisson P, Silver RM. Optimal management strategies for placenta accreta. BJOG. 2009;116(5):648–54.
7. O'Brien JM, Barton JR, Donaldson ES. The management of placenta percreta: conservative and operative strategies. Am J Obstet Gynecol. 1996;175(6):1632–8.
8. Irving F. A study of placenta accreta. Surg Gynecol Obstet. 1937;64:178–200.
9. Allen L, Jauniaux E, Hobson S, Papillon-Smith J, Belfort MA, Diagnosis FPA, et al. FIGO consensus guidelines on placenta accreta spectrum disorders: nonconservative surgical management. Int J Gynaecol Obstet. 2018;140(3):281–90.
10. Society of Gynecologic O, American College of O, Gynecologists, the Society for Maternal-Fetal M, Cahill AG, Beigi R, et al. Placenta Accreta Spectrum. Am J Obstet Gynecol. 2018;219(6):B2–B16.

11. Jauniaux E, Alfirevic Z, Bhide AG, Belfort MA, Burton GJ, Collins SL, et al. Placenta Praevia and placenta Accreta: Diagnosis and management: green-top guideline no. 27a. BJOG. 2019;126(1):e1–e48.
12. Jauniaux E, Kingdom JC, Silver RM. A comparison of recent guidelines in the diagnosis and management of placenta accreta spectrum disorders. Best Pract Res Clin Obstet Gynaecol. 2021;72:102–16.
13. Eller AG, Bennett MA, Sharshiner M, Masheter C, Soisson AP, Dodson M, et al. Maternal morbidity in cases of placenta accreta managed by a multidisciplinary care team compared with standard obstetric care. Obstet Gynecol. 2011;117(2 Pt 1):331–7.
14. Warshak CR, Ramos GA, Eskander R, Benirschke K, Saenz CC, Kelly TF, et al. Effect of predelivery diagnosis in 99 consecutive cases of placenta accreta. Obstet Gynecol. 2010;115(1):65–9.
15. Shamshirsaz AA, Fox KA, Salmanian B, Diaz-Arrastia CR, Lee W, Baker BW, et al. Maternal morbidity in patients with morbidly adherent placenta treated with and without a standardized multidisciplinary approach. Am J Obstet Gynecol. 2015;212(2):218 e1–9.
16. Shainker SA, Coleman B, Timor-Tritsch IE, Bhide A, Bromley B, Cahill AG, et al. Special report of the Society for Maternal-Fetal Medicine Placenta Accreta Spectrum Ultrasound Marker Task Force: consensus on definition of markers and approach to the ultrasound examination in pregnancies at risk for placenta accreta spectrum. Am J Obstet Gynecol. 2021;224(1):B2–B14.
17. D'Antonio F, Iacovella C, Bhide A. Prenatal identification of invasive placentation using ultrasound: systematic review and meta-analysis. Ultrasound Obstet Gynecol. 2013;42(5):509–17.
18. Gielchinsky Y, Mankuta D, Rojansky N, Laufer N, Gielchinsky I, Ezra Y. Perinatal outcome of pregnancies complicated by placenta accreta. Obstet Gynecol. 2004;104(3):527–30.
19. Esakoff TF, Sparks TN, Kaimal AJ, Kim LH, Feldstein VA, Goldstein RB, et al. Diagnosis and morbidity of placenta accreta. Ultrasound Obstet Gynecol. 2011;37(3):324–7.
20. Berkley EM, Abuhamad AZ. Prenatal diagnosis of placenta accreta: is sonography all we need? J Ultrasound Med. 2013;32(8):1345–50.
21. Reddy YS, Ramalaksmi BA, Kumar BD. Lead and trace element levels in placenta, maternal and cord blood: a cross-sectional pilot study. J Obstet Gynaecol Res. 2014;40(12):2184–90.
22. Cali G, Timor-Trisch IE, Palacios-Jaraquemada J, Monteaugudo A, Forlani F, Minneci G, et al. Changes in ultrasonography indicators of abnormally invasive placenta during pregnancy. Int J Gynaecol Obstet. 2018;140(3):319–25.
23. Timor-Tritsch IE, Monteagudo A, Cali G, Vintzileos A, Viscarello R, Al-Khan A, et al. Cesarean scar pregnancy is a precursor of morbidly adherent placenta. Ultrasound Obstet Gynecol. 2014;44(3):346–53.
24. Cali G, Timor-Tritsch IE, Palacios-Jaraquemada J, Monteaugudo A, Buca D, Forlani F, et al. Outcome of cesarean scar pregnancy managed expectantly: systematic review and meta-analysis. Ultrasound Obstet Gynecol. 2018;51(2):169–75.
25. Jauniaux E, Collins S, Burton GJ. Placenta accreta spectrum: pathophysiology and evidence-based anatomy for prenatal ultrasound imaging. Am J Obstet Gynecol. 2018;218(1):75–87.
26. Rac MW, Moschos E, Wells CE, McIntire DD, Dashe JS, Twickler DM. Sonographic findings of morbidly adherent placenta in the first trimester. J Ultrasound Med. 2016;35(2):263–9.
27. Ballas J, Pretorius D, Hull AD, Resnik R, Ramos GA. Identifying sonographic markers for placenta accreta in the first trimester. J Ultrasound Med. 2012;31(11):1835–41.
28. D'Antonio F, Timor-Tritsch IE, Palacios-Jaraquemada J, Monteagudo A, Buca D, Forlani F, et al. First-trimester detection of abnormally invasive placenta in high-risk women: systematic review and meta-analysis. Ultrasound Obstet Gynecol. 2018;51(2):176–83.
29. Cali G, Forlani F, Foti F, Minneci G, Manzoli L, Flacco ME, et al. Diagnostic accuracy of first-trimester ultrasound in detecting abnormally invasive placenta in high-risk women with placenta previa. Ultrasound Obstet Gynecol. 2018;52(2):258–64.
30. Panaiotova J, Tokunaka M, Krajewska K, Zosmer N, Nicolaides KH. Screening for morbidly adherent placenta in early pregnancy. Ultrasound Obstet Gynecol. 2019;53(1):101–6.

31. Bartels HC, Rogers AC, O'Brien D, McVey R, Walsh J, Brennan DJ. Association of implementing a multidisciplinary team approach in the Management of Morbidly Adherent Placenta with Maternal Morbidity and Mortality. Obstet Gynecol. 2018;132(5):1167–76.
32. Pinas Carrillo A, Chandraharan E. Placenta accreta spectrum: risk factors, diagnosis and management with special reference to the triple P procedure. Womens Health (Lond). 2019;15:1745506519878081.
33. Committee Opinion No. 664: refusal of medically recommended treatment during pregnancy. Obstet Gynecol. 2016;127(6):e175–e82.
34. Silver RM. Abnormal placentation: placenta previa, vasa previa, and placenta Accreta. Obstet Gynecol. 2015;126(3):654–68.
35. Walker MG, Allen L, Windrim RC, Kachura J, Pollard L, Pantazi S, et al. Multidisciplinary management of invasive placenta previa. J Obstet Gynaecol Can. 2013;35(5):417–25.
36. Al-Khan A, Gupta V, Illsley NP, Mannion C, Koenig C, Bogomol A, et al. Maternal and fetal outcomes in placenta accreta after institution of team-managed care. Reprod Sci. 2014;21(6):761–71.
37. Jauniaux E, Gronbeck L, Bunce C, Langhoff-Roos J, Collins SL. Epidemiology of placenta previa accreta: a systematic review and meta-analysis. BMJ Open. 2019;9(11):e031193.
38. Wright JD, Herzog TJ, Shah M, Bonanno C, Lewin SN, Cleary K, et al. Regionalization of care for obstetric hemorrhage and its effect on maternal mortality. Obstet Gynecol. 2010;115(6):1194–200.
39. Wright JD, Silver RM, Bonanno C, Gaddipati S, Lu YS, Simpson LL, et al. Practice patterns and knowledge of obstetricians and gynecologists regarding placenta accreta. J Matern Fetal Neonatal Med. 2013;26(16):1602–9.
40. Smulian JC, Pascual AL, Hesham H, Qureshey E, Bijoy Thomas M, Depuy AM, et al. Invasive placental disease: the impact of a multi-disciplinary team approach to management. J Matern Fetal Neonatal Med. 2017;30(12):1423–7.
41. Robinson BK, Grobman WA. Effectiveness of timing strategies for delivery of individuals with placenta previa and accreta. Obstet Gynecol. 2010;116(4):835–42.
42. Norgaard LN, Pinborg A, Lidegaard O, Bergholt T. A Danish national cohort study on neonatal outcome in singleton pregnancies with placenta previa. Acta Obstet Gynecol Scand. 2012;91(5):546–51.
43. Roberts D, Brown J, Medley N, Dalziel SR. Antenatal corticosteroids for accelerating fetal lung maturation for women at risk of preterm birth. Cochrane Database Syst Rev. 2017;3(3):Cd004454.
44. Bose DA, Assel BG, Hill JB, Chauhan SP. Maintenance tocolytics for preterm symptomatic placenta previa: a review. Am J Perinatol. 2011;28(1):45–50.
45. Breymann C, Milman N, Mezzacasa A, Bernard R, Dudenhausen J, investigators F-A. Ferric carboxymaltose vs. oral iron in the treatment of pregnant women with iron deficiency anemia: an international, open-label, randomized controlled trial (FER-ASAP). J Perinat Med. 2017;45(4):443–53.
46. Ruiter L, Eschbach SJ, Burgers M, Rengerink KO, van Pampus MG, Goes BY, et al. Predictors for emergency cesarean delivery in women with placenta Previa. Am J Perinatol. 2016;33(14):1407–14.
47. Pivano A, Alessandrini M, Desbriere R, Agostini A, Opinel P, d'Ercole C, et al. A score to predict the risk of emergency caesarean delivery in women with antepartum bleeding and placenta praevia. Eur J Obstet Gynecol Reprod Biol. 2015;195:173–6.
48. Gyamfi-Bannerman C, Thom EA, Blackwell SC, Tita AT, Reddy UM, Saade GR, et al. Antenatal Betamethasone for Women at Risk for Late Preterm Delivery. N Engl J Med. 2016;374(14):1311–20.
49. Paterson-Brown S, Singh C. Developing a care bundle for the management of suspected placenta accreta. The Obstetrician & Gynaecologist. 2010;12(1):21–7.
50. Ioscovich A, Shatalin D, Butwick AJ, Ginosar Y, Orbach-Zinger S, Weiniger CF. Israeli survey of anesthesia practice related to placenta previa and accreta. Acta Anaesthesiol Scand. 2016;60(4):457–64.

51. Hong JY, Jee YS, Yoon HJ, Kim SM. Comparison of general and epidural anesthesia in elective cesarean section for placenta previa totalis: maternal hemodynamics, blood loss and neonatal outcome. Int J Obstet Anesth. 2003;12(1):12–6.
52. Butwick AJ, Carvalho B, El-Sayed YY. Risk factors for obstetric morbidity in patients with uterine atony undergoing caesarean delivery. Br J Anaesth. 2014;113(4):661–8.
53. Nguyen-Lu N, Carvalho JC, Kingdom J, Windrim R, Allen L, Balki M. Mode of anesthesia and clinical outcomes of patients undergoing cesarean delivery for invasive placentation: a retrospective cohort study of 50 consecutive cases. Can J Anaesth. 2016;63(11):1233–44.
54. Kocaoglu N, Gunusen I, Karaman S, Ergenoglu AM, Firat V. Management of anesthesia for cesarean section in parturients with placenta previa with/without placenta accreta: a retrospective study. Ginekol Pol. 2012;83(2):99–103.
55. Munoz LA, Mendoza GJ, Gomez M, Reyes LE, Arevalo JJ. Anesthetic management of placenta accreta in a low-resource setting: a case series. Int J Obstet Anesth. 2015;24(4):329–34.
56. Taylor NJ, Russell R. Anaesthesia for abnormally invasive placenta: a single-institution case series. Int J Obstet Anesth. 2017;30:10–5.
57. Shamshirsaz AA, Fox KA, Erfani H, Clark SL, Salmanian B, Baker BW, et al. Multidisciplinary team learning in the management of the morbidly adherent placenta: outcome improvements over time. Am J Obstet Gynecol. 2017;216(6):612 e1–5.
58. Committee opinion no. 529: placenta accreta. Obstet Gynecol. 2012;120(1):207–11.
59. Matsubara S, Kuwata T, Usui R, Watanabe T, Izumi A, Ohkuchi A, et al. Important surgical measures and techniques at cesarean hysterectomy for placenta previa accreta. Acta Obstet Gynecol Scand. 2013;92(4):372–7.
60. Tam Tam KB, Dozier J, Martin JN Jr. Approaches to reduce urinary tract injury during management of placenta accreta, increta, and percreta: a systematic review. J Matern Fetal Neonatal Med. 2012;25(4):329–34.
61. Norris BL, Everaerts W, Posma E, Murphy DG, Umstad MP, Costello AJ, et al. The urologist's role in multidisciplinary management of placenta percreta. BJU Int. 2016;117(6):961–5.
62. Camuzcuoglu A, Vural M, Hilali NG, Incebiyik A, Yuce HH, Kucuk A, et al. Surgical management of 58 patients with placenta praevia percreta. Wien Klin Wochenschr. 2016;128(9–10):360–6.
63. Walker MG, Pollard L, Talati C, Carvalho JC, Allen LM, Kachura J, et al. Obstetric and Anaesthesia checklists for the management of morbidly adherent placenta. J Obstet Gynaecol Can. 2016;38(11):1015–23.
64. Simonazzi G, Bisulli M, Saccone G, Moro E, Marshall A, Berghella V. Tranexamic acid for preventing postpartum blood loss after cesarean delivery: a systematic review and meta-analysis of randomized controlled trials. Acta Obstet Gynecol Scand. 2016;95(1):28–37.
65. Lakshmi SD, Abraham R. Role of prophylactic tranexamic acid in reducing blood loss during elective caesarean section: a randomized controlled study. J Clin Diagn Res. 2016;10(12):QC17–21.
66. Ray I, Bhattacharya R, Chakraborty S, Bagchi C, Mukhopadhyay S. Role of intravenous tranexamic acid on caesarean blood loss: A prospective randomised study. J Obstet Gynaecol India. 2016;66(Suppl 1):347–52.
67. Shah D, Chudasama D, Patel D, Vyas D, Parikh D, Dodiya D, et al. Placenta Accreta spectrum (pas) disorders: a 10-year study at tertiary care center, Ahmedabad, western India. Int J Clinical Obstet Gynaecol. 2020;4:161–6.
68. McDonnell NJ, Kennedy D, Long LJ, Gallagher-Swann MC, Paech MJ. The development and implementation of an obstetric cell salvage service. Anaesth Intensive Care. 2010;38(3):492–9.
69. Elagamy A, Abdelaziz A, Ellaithy M. The use of cell salvage in women undergoing cesarean hysterectomy for abnormal placentation. Int J Obstet Anesth. 2013;22(4):289–93.
70. Lew E, Tagore S. Implementation of an obstetric cell salvage service in a tertiary women's hospital. Singap Med J. 2015;56(8):445–9.
71. Sentilhes L, Kayem G, Chandraharan E, Palacios-Jaraquemada J, Jauniaux E. FIGO consensus guidelines on placenta accreta spectrum disorders: conservative management. Int J Gynaecol Obstet. 2018;140(3):291–8.

72. Selman AE. Caesarean hysterectomy for placenta praevia/accreta using an approach via the pouch of Douglas. BJOG. 2016;123(5):815–9.
73. Belfort MA, Shamshirsaz AA, Fox KA. A technique to positively identify the vaginal fornices during complicated postpartum hysterectomy. Am J Obstet Gynecol. 2017;217(2):222.e1–3.
74. Belfort MA, Shamshiraz AA, Fox K. Minimizing blood loss at cesarean-hysterectomy for placenta previa percreta. Am J Obstet Gynecol. 2017;216(1):78.e1–2.
75. Verspyck E, Douysset X, Roman H, Marret S, Marpeau L. Transecting versus avoiding incision of the anterior placenta previa during cesarean delivery. Int J Gynaecol Obstet. 2015;128(1):44–7.
76. Khan M, Sachdeva P, Arora R, Bhasin S. Conservative management of morbidly adherant placenta - a case report and review of literature. Placenta. 2013;34(10):963–6.
77. C BL, Coker A, Lawal AH, Abu J, Cowen MJ. The B-lynch surgical technique for the control of massive postpartum haemorrhage: an alternative to hysterectomy? Five cases reported. Br J Obstet Gynaecol. 1997;104(3):372–5.
78. Yoong W, Ridout A, Memtsa M, Stavroulis A, Aref-Adib M, Ramsay-Marcelle Z, et al. Application of uterine compression suture in association with intrauterine balloon tamponade ('uterine sandwich') for postpartum hemorrhage. Acta Obstet Gynecol Scand. 2012;91(1):147–51.
79. El Gelany SA, Abdelraheim AR, Mohammed MM, Gad El-Rab MT, Yousef AM, Ibrahim EM, et al. The cervix as a natural tamponade in postpartum hemorrhage caused by placenta previa and placenta previa accreta: a prospective study. BMC Pregnancy Childbirth. 2015;15:295.
80. Huang G, Zhou R, Hu Y. A new suture technique for cesarean delivery complicated by hemorrhage in cases of placenta previa accreta. Int J Gynaecol Obstet. 2014;124(3):262–3.
81. Kaplanoğlu M, Kaplanoğlu DK, Koyuncu O. A different approach to placenta previa accreta: intrauterine gauze compress combined B-Lynch uterine compression suture. Clin Exp Obstet Gynecol. 2015;42(1):53–6.
82. Shazly SA, Badee AY, Ali MK. The use of multiple 8 compression suturing as a novel procedure to preserve fertility in patients with placenta accreta: case series. Aust N Z J Obstet Gynaecol. 2012;52(4):395–9.
83. Esakoff TF, Handler SJ, Granados JM, Caughey AB. PAMUS: placenta accreta management across the United States. J Matern Fetal Neonatal Med. 2012;25(6):761–5.
84. ACOG Practice Bulletin No. 84: prevention of deep vein thrombosis and pulmonary embolism. Obstet Gynecol. 2007;110(2 Pt 1):429–40.
85. Bratzler DW, Dellinger EP, Olsen KM, Perl TM, Auwaerter PG, Bolon MK, et al. Clinical practice guidelines for antimicrobial prophylaxis in surgery. Am J Health Syst Pharm. 2013;70(3):195–283.
86. Shakur H, Beaumont D, Pavord S, Gayet-Ageron A, Ker K, Mousa HA. Antifibrinolytic drugs for treating primary postpartum haemorrhage. Cochrane Database Syst Rev. 2018;2(2):Cd012964.
87. Arendas K, Lortie KJ, Singh SS. Delayed laparoscopic management of placenta increta. J Obstet Gynaecol Can. 2012;34(2):186–9.
88. Smith DD, Perez-Delboy A, Burke WM, Tergas AI. Buttock necrosis after uterine artery embolization for delayed hysterectomy in placenta Percreta. Case Rep Obstet Gynecol. 2016;2016:6921280.
89. Rupley DM, Tergas AI, Palmerola KL, Burke WM. Robotically assisted delayed total laparoscopic hysterectomy for placenta percreta. Gynecol Oncol Rep. 2016;17:53–5.
90. Publications Committee SfM-FM, Belfort MA. Placenta accreta. Am J Obstet Gynecol. 2010;203(5):430–9.

Chapter 15
Management of Placenta Accreta Spectrum in the Second Trimester

Omima T. Taha, Maryam Abdelkarim, Nourah Al Qahtani, and Ayman S. Dawood

Introduction

Placental accreta, previously known as morbidly adherent placenta, was first described by Irving et al. in 1937 [1]. This term was first used to describe placental invasion beyond the decidua. Placenta accreta spectrum (PAS) is a more recent terminology, proposed by the International Federation of Gynecology and Obstetrics (FIGO), that includes different degrees of placenta invasion including accreta, increta, and percreta [2].

Incidence of PAS has significantly increased from 0.8 in 1000 deliveries in the 1980s to 3 in 1000 deliveries in the last decade. The rising trend of PAS has been primarily attributed to global increase in cesarean section (CS) rate [3]. PAS is a life-threatening condition owing to potential massive obstetrical hemorrhage, which increases risk of peripartum hysterectomy, maternal morbidity, and mortality, which reaches up to 7% in some regions [4, 5, 6]. Currently, incidence of second trimester pregnancy termination, secondary to PAS, has risen from 0.04 [7] to 2.3% [8]. Second trimester termination for PAS aims at reducing risk of massive hemorrhage

O. T. Taha (✉)
Obstetrics and Gynecology Department, Faculty of Medicine, Suez Canal University, Ismailia, Egypt

M. Abdelkarim
Obstetrics and Gynecology Department, Faculty of Medicine, Alexandria University, Alexandria, Egypt

N. Al Qahtani
Obstetrics and Gynecology Department, Imam Abdulrahman Bin Faisal University, Dammam, Kingdom of Saudi Arabia

A. S. Dawood
Obstetrics and Gynecology Department, Faculty of Medicine, Tanta University, Tanta, Egypt

S. A. Shazly, A. A. Nassr (eds.), *Placenta Accreta Spectrum*,
https://doi.org/10.1007/978-3-031-10347-6_15

and spontaneous uterine rupture requiring hysterectomy compared to conventional third trimester management [9–11].

Pathophysiology

The most contributing risk factors for development of PAS are number of previous CSs and placental site. When CS scar is combined with placental implantation in the lower uterine segment, risk of accretion is substantially high, reaching up to 61% in women with previous three CSs [12]. The presence of uterine scar leads to defective decidualization, which precipitates abnormal invasion of the placenta in ensuing pregnancy. Similarly, any disruption of the endometrial lining carries a varying risk of PAS [13]. PAS is classified into placental accreta, increta, and percreta according to the extent of myometrial invasion. Placental accreta, which is the least invasive subtype of PAS, presents the most prevalent form, and it counts for 75% of cases [14]. In general, the pattern of placental proliferation and invasion mimics neoplastic disorders. Both conditions share the capability of overcoming the immune system, activating invasion, and inducing angiogenesis [15]. These mechanisms are precipitated by defective decidua basalis, which results from defective endometrial-myometrial interface due to previous uterine scarring [16], abnormal remodeling of maternal vasculature, and marked trophoblastic invasion [17]. The role of different surgical techniques of uterine incision closure, in pathogenesis of PAS, remains controversial [18]. One of these technical variants is single versus double closure of the incision; single-layer closure of uterine incision with continuous locked sutures was associated with subsequent thinner uterine thickness in some studies [19]. However, other studies did not conclude any significant difference in scar thickness among women who had single-layer versus double-layer closure of uterine incision [20]. Overall, there are currently no recommendations that would support a particular technique to close the uterus for the purpose of preventing PAS, and further research is warranted to recognize more preventable risk factors, if any, to reduce incidence of PAS in contemporary population.

Diagnosis

In women with prior CS, sonographers performing first-trimester ultrasound should be conscious of the features of cesarean scar pregnancy (CSP), which is currently considered by many experts as the precursor of PAS [1]. Most sonographic signs can be detected between 11th and 14th weeks of gestation and early in the second trimester, which coincides with routine dating scan, unless earlier scans are indicated due to suspicious symptoms [2].

PAS is progressive in nature, and the course of invasion may progress starting at the 28th week of gestation. Thus, serial ultrasound scans may be required to define depth and extent of the invasion and determine management [3, 4]. Nevertheless, PAS is an intraoperative diagnosis, confirmed by postpartum histopathological examination, and eventual management may be altered by intraoperative findings. Nevertheless, current imaging modalities, accompanied by growing experience in antepartum diagnosis of PAS, have enhanced antepartum diagnostic accuracy and permitted preoperative counseling and management plan with high level of confidence. Highest diagnostic accuracy can be achieved by combining transabdominal and transvaginal ultrasound approaches, adjusting machine settings, and considering appropriate gestational age at scanning. Furthermore, sonographic examination while the bladder is full and correct insonation angle of the probe facilitate assessment of extent of invasion [5]. Ultrasound yields a sensitivity of 90.7% and specificity of 96.9% for diagnosis of PAS associated with low placental site. However, it has a limited role in diagnosing non-previa PAS disorders, and negative predictive value may reach as high as 84% [6, 7].

In the second trimester, sonographic findings, suggestive of PAS disorders, include abnormal utero-placental interface (clear zone), extreme thinning of the underlying myometrium, and placenta lacunae. These signs may be present in low-risk non-PAS pregnancies. However, their presence, in high-risk women, yields the highest sensitivity of all grayscale 2D markers. Sonographic assessment also includes color Doppler assessment of uterovesical interface, which may reveal bridging vessels and interruption of bladder wall in women with PAS [8]. In many occasions, visual extension of placental tissue into the uterus and/or bladder (placental bulge) may raise suspicion of placenta percreta [9]. More recently, "rail sign" was described as a Doppler marker of PAS. This sign refers to sonographic appearance of two parallel vessels with multiple connecting vessels at placenta-bladder interface and is suspicious of placenta percreta. The sign was also associated with increased risk of massive blood loss exceeding 2000 ml [10].

In diagnosis of PAS, magnetic resonance imaging (MRI) is not superior to conventional ultrasound. Specifically, MRI is rather complementary, when ultrasound is technical restricted such as when placenta is posteriorly localized or in women with high body mass index. In these cases, the pelvis can be clear visualized, and extent of invasion can be determined with offline revaluation [11, 12].

MRI features of PAS are usually classified into direct and indirect signs. Indirect signs embrace placental heterogeneity; T2-hypo-intense intraparenchymal dark bands, hypervascularity with tortuous, disorganized intraparenchymal vessels, and proliferated pelvic and retro-uterine veins [13]. The "recess sign," described by Sato et al., refers to the presence of a wedge-shaped placental deformity with contraction of the placental surface and outer rim of the uterus, accompanied by a T2 dark band. In the original study, this finding was highly associated with abnormal placental invasion (increta, percreta) [14].

The direct signs include disordered normal myometrial trilaminar signal with/without directly visualized invasion, focal bulge, especially at the lower uterine segment, and directly visualized extrauterine placental extension. The more severe the case of PAS (increta, percreta), the more disrupted the outline of the uterus. Therefore, instead of the classic inverted pear-shaped uterus, the lower segment becomes broader than the fundus [15]. Invasion of nearby pelvic structures such as bladder dome or rectal invasion is suspicious of placenta percreta [13, 16].

Management

Proper management of PAS can be initiated by antenatal diagnosis, which permits multidisciplinary planning and referral to specialized centers and, hence, lowers risk of maternal mortality and morbidity [17] . Ideally, diagnosis of PAS should be suspected in the second trimester. This facilitates early referral and establishment of care, optimization of maternal condition (such as correction of anemia), and protection against unplanned deliveries. Women at higher risk of preterm labor may be offered antenatal steroids between 23 and 34 weeks of gestation and are likely to be hospitalized in the second or early third trimester until delivery. Additional ultrasound at 32 to 34 weeks should be offered to verify placental location and assess invasion prior to delivery planning [18].

Second-Trimester Termination

There is no consensus on second-trimester pregnancy termination for PAS disorders, and data on termination techniques are sparse in the literature. In fact, most evidence is derived from case reports of termination for other indications such as concurrent fetal anomalies, preterm prelabor rupture of membranes (PPROM), or intrauterine fetal death (IUFD). In many reported cases, induction of labor was conducted to deliver the fetus, followed by a trial to separate the placenta. Surgical intervention was confined to cases where placental delivery was not possible and was either by en bloc hysterectomy or focal resection and other conservative techniques [19].

Cui et al. studied 29 patients with PAS disorders who underwent termination of pregnancy in the second trimester. After delivery, morbidly adherent placentas were left in situ and adjuvant interventions were considered including uterine artery embolization, misoprostol, methotrexate, or Chinese traditional medicines. Uterine preservation was achieved in 26 cases out of 29 [20] . On the other hand, Matsuzaki et al. reported the use of prostaglandin E1 (gemeprost) for pregnancy termination in a 20-week pregnant woman with PPROM, which was complicated by massive hemorrhage and subsequent hysterectomy [21]. Nakayama et al. reported 11 patients: 4 underwent dilatation and curettage and 7 had gemeprost termination safely with no significant difference in mean intraoperative blood loss. However, these cases were diagnosed with placenta previa and diagnosis of PAS was not made [22].

Scheduled Hysterotomy

Ou et al. conducted a retrospective study on 28 cases with second-trimester termination of pregnancy in the presence of PAS. Uterine preservation was achieved in all cases. In this cohort, eight women were antenatally diagnosed with PAS and were delivered through hysterotomy. The remaining 20 women were diagnosed postnatally and were managed by leaving placenta in situ. Adjuvant treatment was given to the patients and the placenta passed out within 43.5 (7–102) days after termination. One case of uterine infection was reported [23]. Similarly, Tocce et al. concluded that scheduled hysterotomy for termination of pregnancy in the second trimester, if PAS is suspected, is a recommended strategy [24].

Tian et al. published a case series of women with placenta previa and scarred uterus, who underwent termination/induction of labor in second and third trimesters. These women were managed by mifepristone, extra-amniotic ethacridine lactate, and uterine artery embolization for women with complete placenta previa. This approach was successful in 83.3% of cases. Interestingly, success was not related to age, parity, number, or time of prior hysterectomies. However, failure was related to time interval between current pregnancy and previous surgery [25]. Hu et al. included 51 patients who underwent pregnancy termination in the second trimester, retrospectively. All patients had prior CS with current placenta previa accreta. Thirty-one cases received mifepristone and extra-amniotic Rivanol medical termination, and only one patient was converted to hysterotomy. The remaining 20 women underwent planned hysterotomy [26]. Of note, some of the abovementioned studies used unestablished treatment options such as Rivanol and ethacridine, which may be less known to contemporary medicine and are likely supported by local authorities. Accordingly, implementation of these strategies may be clinically and ethically challenging.

Peripartum Hysterectomy

This approach may be considered in elective environment, especially when future fertility is not desired, or in emergency situations due to significant hemorrhage [27]. Compared to third trimester delivery, second-trimester termination permits the privilege of considering non-laparotomy options, including laparoscopy and robotic-assisted surgery, due to uterine size. Boes et al. reported a 20-week pregnant patient, diagnosed with PPROM and IUFD, who was successfully managed by robotic-assisted hysterectomy. Similarly, the same procedure was reported by Elfeky et al., which was successfully performed to manage a 16-week pregnancy complicated with placenta increta [28, 29].

Leaving Placenta In Situ

As mentioned earlier in this chapter, leaving the placenta in situ was considered in few studies to permit vaginal delivery of second trimester PAS and when PAS is accidently discovered after delivery of the fetus if there is no significant bleeding. Similar to third trimester management of PAS, leaving placenta in situ is not without risk, and this approach is associated with concerns on risk of infection, long follow-up, and patient compliance. A thorough counseling should be considered and managing team should be familiar with this approach.

Conclusion

Evidence on second-trimester termination of pregnancy in women with suspected PAS is limited. Therefore, management is prone to institutional and surgeons' preference. PAS is commonly missed in women undergoing early termination of pregnancy and is first diagnosed intra- or postpartum. In addition to conventional management of PAS, women in the second trimester may be offered minimally invasive procedures for planned hysterectomy. Women who desire to preserve their fertility may be offered planned hysterotomy with a trial of uterine preservation. Termination of pregnancy through vaginal route was also reported in the literature. However, clinical outcomes are unpredictable, and risk of massive bleeding and emergency surgery should not be underestimated. Therefore, this approach is the most controversial unless diagnosis of PAS was not made antenatally. In these circumstances, retained placenta would warrant further management depending on amount of bleeding and hemodynamic stability. Women who are actively bleeding should undergo emergency surgery. However, management of those who experience mild or no bleeding is less evident and it should be determined by patient and obstetrician's preference in concordance with institutional experience and internal policies.

References

1. Timor-Tritsch IE, et al. Early first-trimester transvaginal ultrasound is indicated in pregnancy after previous Cesarean delivery: should it be mandatory? Ultrasound Obstet Gynecol. 2019;54(2):156–63.
2. Reddy UM, et al. Fetal imaging: executive summary of a joint Eunice Kennedy Shriver National Institute of child health and human development, Society for Maternal-Fetal medicine, American Institute of ultrasound in medicine, American College of obstetricians and Gynecologists, American College of radiology, Society for pediatric radiology, and society of radiologists in ultrasound fetal imaging workshop. J Ultrasound Med. 2014;210(5):387–97.
3. Calì G, et al. Changes in ultrasonography indicators of abnormally invasive placenta during pregnancy. Int J Gynaecol Obstet. 2018;140(3):319–25.

4. Comstock CH, et al. Sonographic detection of placenta accreta in the second and third trimesters of pregnancy. Am J Obstet Gynecol. 2004;190(4):1135–40.
5. Chantraine F, Collins SLJCO, Reports G. Prenatal ultrasound imaging for placenta Accreta Spectrum (PAS): a Practical Guide. Curr Obstet Gynecol. 2019;8(3):86–93.
6. D'antonio F, et al. Prenatal identification of invasive placentation using ultrasound: systematic review and meta-analysis. Ultrasound Obstet Gynecol. 2013;42(5):509–17.
7. Kocher MR, et al. Diagnosis of abnormally invasive posterior placentation: the role of MR imaging. Radiology Case Reports. 2017;12(2):295–9.
8. Philips J, et al. Prevalence of sonographic markers of placenta accreta spectrum in low-risk pregnancies. Am J Perinatol. 2019;36(08):733–80.
9. Jauniaux E, et al. Accreta placentation: a systematic review of prenatal ultrasound imaging and grading of villous invasiveness. Am J Obstet Gynecol. 2016;215(6):712–21.
10. Shih J-C, et al. The "rail sign": an ultrasound finding in placenta accreta spectrum indicating deep villous invasion and adverse outcomes. Am J Obstet Gynecol. 2021;225(3):292.e1–292.e17.
11. Morlando M, Collins S. Placenta accreta spectrum disorders: challenges, risks, and management strategies. Int J Womens Health. 2020;12:1033.
12. Einerson BD, et al. Magnetic resonance imaging is often misleading when used as an adjunct to ultrasound in the management of placenta accreta spectrum disorders. Am J Obstet Gynecol. 2018;218(6):618.e1–7.
13. Brown BP, Meyers ML. Placental magnetic resonance imaging Part II: placenta accreta spectrum. Pediatr Radiol. 2020;50(2):275–84.
14. Sato T, et al. Placental recess accompanied by a T2 dark band: a new finding for diagnosing placental invasion. Abdom Radiol (NY). 2017;42(8):2146–53.
15. D'antonio F, et al. Prenatal identification of invasive placentation using magnetic resonance imaging: systematic review and meta-analysis. Ultrasound Obstet Gynecol. 2014;44(1):8–16.
16. Knight JC, et al. A comprehensive severity score for the morbidly adherent placenta: combining ultrasound and magnetic resonance imaging. Pediatr Radiol. 2018;48(13):1945–54.
17. Silver RM, et al. Center of excellence for placenta accreta. Am J Obstet Gynecol. 2015;212(5):561–8.
18. Collins SL, et al. Evidence-based guidelines for the management of abnormally invasive placenta: recommendations from the International Society for Abnormally Invasive Placenta. Am J Obstet Gynecol. 2019;220(6):511–26.
19. Ruano R, et al. Second-and third-trimester therapeutic terminations of pregnancy in cases with complete placenta previa–does feticide decrease postdelivery maternal hemorrhage? Fetal Diagn Ther. 2004;19(6):475–8.
20. Cui R, et al. Management strategies for patients with placenta accreta spectrum disorders who underwent pregnancy termination in the second trimester: a retrospective study. BMC Pregnancy Childbirth. 2018;18(1):1–8.
21. Matsuzaki S, et al. A case report and literature review of Midtrimester termination of pregnancy complicated by placenta Previa and placenta Accreta. American Journal of Perinatology Reports. 2014;05(01):e006–11.
22. Nakayama D, et al. Effect of placenta previa on blood loss in second-trimester abortion by labor induction using gemeprost. Contraception. 2007;75(3):238–40.
23. Ou J, et al. Management of patients with placenta accreta spectrum disorders who underwent pregnancy terminations in the second trimester: a retrospective study. Eur J Obstet Gynecol Reprod Biol. 2019;242:109–13.
24. Tocce K, Thomas VW, Teal S. Scheduled hysterectomy for second-trimester abortion in a patient with placenta accreta. Obstet Gynecol. 2009;113(2):568–70.
25. Tian J-S, et al. Risk factors of pregnancy termination at second and third trimester in women with scarred uterus and placenta previa. J Zhejiang Univ (Med Sci). 2015;44(3):247–52.

26. Hu Q, et al. Clinical analysis of second-trimester pregnancy termination after previous caesarean delivery in 51 patients with placenta previa and placenta accreta spectrum: a retrospective study. BMC Pregnancy Childbirth. 2021;21(1):1–11.
27. Matsuzaki S, et al. A case report and literature review of midtrimester termination of pregnancy complicated by placenta previa and placenta accreta. AJP Rep. 2015;5(01):e6–e11.
28. Boes S, et al. Peripartum robotic-assisted laparoscopic hysterectomy after second-trimester pregnancy loss with placenta increta. Obstet Gynecol. 2013;122(2):440–4.
29. Elfeky A, et al. Elective robotic hysterectomy for placenta accreta spectrum in the second trimester: case report. Int J Surg Case Rep. 2020;72:361–4.

Chapter 16
Long-Term Outcomes of Conservative Management of PAS: Long-Term Sequences and Impact on Future Pregnancies

Mahmoud A. Abdel-Aleem

Introduction

Placenta accreta spectrum disorder (PAS) comprises placenta accreta, increta, and percreta, which are adhesive disorders of placentation with different levels of severity [1]. The term "placenta accreta" is a histopathologic term for a condition first described in 1937 by obstetrician Frederick C. Irving and pathologist Arthur T. Hertig at the Boston Lying-in Hospital [2]. They described 18 new cases of placenta accreta presenting with "the abnormal adherence of the afterbirth in whole or in parts to the underlying uterine wall." They picked the attention to the major postpartum hemorrhage during the attempts to remove the placenta. Hysterectomy was done to control the bleeding in 14 cases.

Its course and the rate of complications are difficult to be determined except intraoperative, but in a good proportion of cases it has a gloomy prognosis. It may lead to high maternal morbidity and mortality due to its inherent wild killing hemorrhage, unforeseen cesarean hysterectomy, and other complexities resulting from abnormal invasion of the placenta into adjacent organs.

Notwithstanding the enormous improvement made in the prevention of maternal death due to obstetric bleeding caused by atony, genital laceration, and coagulopathies since the first edition of the *Williams Obstetrics* textbook was published in 1903, maternal mortality and morbidity due to PAS are greatly amplified during the twenty-first century [3]. Obstetricians are confronted with a rising number of cases making it one of the most important currently happening obstetric catastrophes.

In parallel with an increasing rate of cesarean delivery, the prevalence of PAS has tripled over the last 30 years, from 0.1% of deliveries in the 1980s to 0.3% [4]. This rising prevalence is accompanied by an alarming risk of maternal deaths.

M. A. Abdel-Aleem (✉)
Department of Obstetrics and Gynecology, Assiut University, Assiut, Egypt

S. A. Shazly, A. A. Nassr (eds.), *Placenta Accreta Spectrum*,
https://doi.org/10.1007/978-3-031-10347-6_16

The lack of randomized clinical trials makes the optimal management of PAS disorders remains undefined and is determined by the facility to diagnose invasive placentation preoperatively, surgeon expertise, depth of villous invasion, and presenting symptoms.

Until recently, elective caesarean hysterectomy was an accepted approach to hemostasis in patients with PAS, but its concomitant morbidities affect both the culture and the female own insights about menstruation and future fertility [5]. Consequently, more conservative, uterus-preserving approaches have been practiced. Each technique has its one benefits and limitations and of course its applicability in whichever surgical scenario.

To choose between hysterectomy and conservative management for placenta accrete isn't an easy decision to make. On one hand, to reduce maternal morbidity and mortality, elective cesarean hysterectomy in a tertiary care hospital with a multidisciplinary care team deems to be the safest and most common treatment for cases diagnosed before delivery. However, the decision of hysterectomy for placenta accreta may be difficult to make. In these cases, systematic manual separation of the placenta from the uterine wall is usually performed. In other cases, excision of a part of the uterine wall with re-suturing looks logical and effective [5].

A great and common obligatory indication for leaving placenta in situ is "percreta" variety with involvement of nearby organs such as the urinary bladder, bowel, or any other pelvic structure [6].

An Old, Long, but Meaningful Story

The following is a case report of placenta accreta or increta that was treated conservatively with no harmful effects, 1 year after the patient had a normal delivery with a normal third stage.

A patient, aged 31 years, had been under treatment for infertility. She got pregnant for the first time but aborted at 22 cm fetus on August 16, 1946. All efforts to express the placenta failed both with and without anesthesia. Palpation of the uterine cavity by both the operator and his assistant revealed no line of cleavage of the placenta. It was impossible to determine where the placenta ended and the uterine wall began. Because there was practically no bleeding, it was decided to follow a conservative course, and the patient again was returned to bed; she was kept in the hospital for 1 week under medical treatment. No serious bleeding nor evidence of infection developed so she was transferred home. She remained in bed at home for 3 weeks, during which time the uterus drained a bloody purulent lochia. Her only complaint was cramps and pains in the legs, especially at night. Two weeks after the delivery, the fundus was not palpable abdominally. From the fourth to eighth week postpartum, the uterine drainage was of a bright bloody character and very moderate in amount. All discharge stopped on October 10, 1946. She had her next pregnancy diagnosed on February 1, 1947. This time, her pregnancy was essentially normal throughout, and she was delivered of a normal infant on September 24, 1947, after an 11-hour labor. A grossly normal placenta was delivered 2 minutes later by simple expression. Postpartum bleeding and the entire puerperium were normal [7]. This story implies the success of conservative management of placenta accreta with a good outcome thereafter.

Definitions and Problems

A general dilemma in studies on PAS is the definition of this condition: some studies are established on prenatal imaging criteria, some on clinical characteristics, and others on histopathology [8].

Conservative management of PAS is defined as removal of the placenta with uterine preservation [8]. However, this term is used also to describe "leaving placenta in situ without touching it." Conservative management, intentionally leaving the placenta in situ 7: after delivery, no effort is made to remove the placenta; the placenta is left in situ for either spontaneous reabsorption (i.e., for fertility-sparing management) 8 or planned delayed hysterectomy (an option often used in placenta percreta with the aim of reducing surgical complexity).

Another term is "successful conservative treatment" as defined by uterine preservation, i.e., the absence of either immediate or delayed hysterectomy due to PAS [9].

In a large multicenter study, it was shown that this conservative treatment (leaving the placenta in situ untouched) could preserve the uterus in 78.4% [95% confidence interval (CI), 71.4 84.4%] of women, with a severe maternal morbidity rate of only 6% (95% CI, 2.9–10.7%) [9].

Most publications on the PAS including reviews consist of a highly variable blend of women with placenta accreta, increta, and percreta getting on to a little bit biased conclusions [10].

Lines of Conservative Management [5]

Conservative management of both abnormally adherent (placenta accreta) and invasive placenta (placenta increta and percreta) defines all procedures that aim to avoid peripartum hysterectomy and its related morbidity and consequences.

A variety of conservative options for the management of PAS disorders have evolved, each with varying rates of success and peripartum and secondary complications [10].

In a recent systematic review and meta-analysis of the outcome of placenta previa accreta diagnosed prenatally, 208 out of 232 (89.7%) cases had an elective or emergent cesarean hysterectomy [11].

A list of conservative management lines are (Table 16.1):

1. Conservative surgical management of PAS with removal of placenta (the extirpative approach).

Table 16.1 Studies addressing different lines of management of PAS

Reference	Conservative (local excision)	Leaving placenta in situ	Hysterectomy
[12]	37 (47%)	15 (19%)	27 (34%)
[10]	17 (14%)	36 (30%)	66 (56%)
{van Beekhuizen, 2021 #242}	26 women (5.9%)	In 48 women (10.8%), of those, 20 (41.7%) had a delayed hysterectomy	252 women (57.0%) with a repeat laparotomy in 20 (7.9%) due to complications
{Durukan, 2021 #326}	23/148	83/148 plus use of Bakri balloon	42/ 148

2. Leaving the placenta in situ (expectant approach).
3. One-step en bloc focal resection of underlying myometrium: currently the most trendy operation. It is done for a focal PAS. At cesarean section, the transverse incision in the uterine wall is placed cranially above the abnormally invasive part of the placenta and the baby is delivered. The placenta and affected myometrium are then removed and the uterus is closed [13].
4. Triple P procedure: suturing around the accreta area after resection. Future pregnancy isn't recommended {Teixidor Vinas, 2015 #506}.
5. Adjuvant techniques: used as an adjunct to main line of management to help in reducing the impact of blood loss:

    (a) Uterine devascularization.
    (b) Use of uterine hemostatic sutures.
    (c) Use of Bakri balloon with excision of uterine wall {Ustunyurt, 2020 #295}.
    (d) Balloon occlusion of aorta, common iliac or internal iliac artery {Jauniaux, 2022 #160}{Matsubara, 2018 #442} {Matsubara, 2021 #141}{Peng, 2020 #324}.
    (e) Uterine artery embolization: Studies examining pelvic artery embolization in combination with conservative management have reported success rates of 60%–95% [9].
    (f) Adjuvant use of methotrexate has been reported with conflicting opinions between advocates and opponents. Its use is hypothesized to add to the success of conservative management by accelerating the autolysis of the placenta that was left in situ.

Long-Term Complications

Intrauterine Synechiae

Being affecting both menstrual pattern (amenorrhea/ hypomenorrhea) and fertility potential, it is an important point that should be discussed with a patient who deemed to undergo conservative management for PAS.

Of the 96 women successfully contacted at follow-up, 88 had resumed menstruation. Severe intrauterine synechiae (stage III) were identified during office hysteroscopy in eight women with amenorrhea. One of these eight women declined further treatment; hysteroscopic treatment of the synechiae was successful for six of the remaining seven women {Sentilhes, 2010 #488}.

Synechiae rates did not differ significantly according to the type of conservative treatment: uterine compression suture [0/7 (0%) versus 8/89 (9.0%); P. 0.99], pelvic arterial embolization [1/41 (2.4%) versus 7/55 (12.7.0%); $P < 0.13$], or vessel ligation [1/24 (4.2%) versus 7/72 (9.7%); $P < 0.67$]. There were 12 other women, 5 complaining of decreased menstrual flow and 7 for other routine reasons, who also underwent outpatient hysteroscopy, which was normal in all cases.

Impaired Fertility

A large series conducted by Sentilhes and his group implied that successful conservative treatment for placenta accreta does not appear to affect women's subsequent fertility or obstetric outcome but that the risk of recurrence of placenta accreta during future deliveries is high [9]. They described a series of 167 patients who underwent conservative management for PAS.

Negative Impact on Subsequent Pregnancies (Fig. 16.1)

In their analysis, they ended with 96 patients with data available. Twenty-four cases got pregnant (with a total of 34 pregnancies) {Sentilhes, 2010 #482} The long-term obstetric profile is described in the following chart.

Of the 27 women who wanted more children, 24 (88.9%) had 34 pregnancies with a mean time to conception of 17.3 months (range: 2–48 months). All deliveries resulted in healthy babies born after 34 weeks of gestation.

(a) *Maternal impact {Kabiri, 2014 #49}*

   (i) No increased risk of placenta previa, gestational DM, hypertensive disorders, placental abruption, cesarean delivery or postpartum infection.
   (ii) Increased risk of second trimester bleeding (OR 9.37 95% CI 2.2–38.8).
   (iii) Increased risk of placenta accreta (RR 12.13 95% CI 4.95–29.69). The wide confidence interval points to weak precision.
   (iv) Increased risk of early postpartum hemorrhage (RR 3.29 95% CI 1.43–7.53) {Kabiri, 2014 #49}. In another study, it occurred on four [19.0% (95% CI, 5.4–41.9%)] occasions, related to placenta accreta in three cases and to uterine atony in one [9].
   (v) Increased risk of manual removal of placenta (aRR 6.92, 95% CI 3.81–12.55) {Baldwin, 2020 #26}.

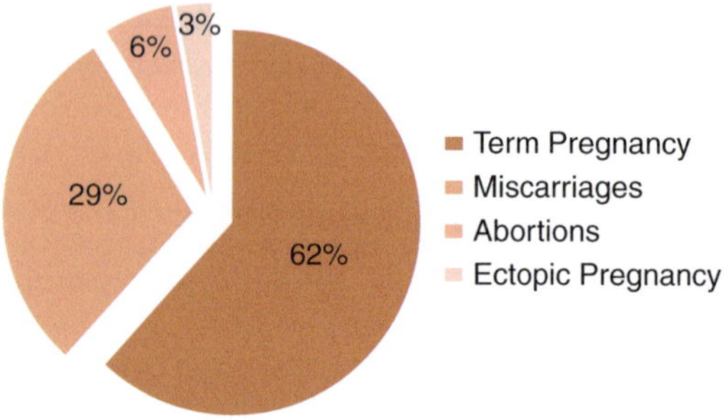

Fig. 16.1 Obstetric outcomes of pregnancies after conservative management of placenta accreta spectrum

(vi) Increased risk of rupture uterus, maternal blood transfusion, wound infection, intensive care unit admission {Eshkoli, 2013 #56}.
(vii) Increased risk of cesarean hysterectomy {Eshkoli, 2013 #56}.

(b) *Fetal/neonatal impact*

(i) No increased risk twin pregnancy, intrauterine fetal death
(ii) Conflicting results on the risk of preterm birth, ranging from no increased risk to preterm birth (aRR 1.43, 95% CI 1.03–1.98), with lower risk of small for gestational age (aRR 0.64, 95% CI 0.43–0.96), compared with similar-risk births

Possible Effect of Arterial Embolization {Sentilhes, 2010 #507}

Analysis was done for 68 cases. Among the 15 women who complained of amenorrhea or hypomenorrhea, synechia was found in all those who opted to undergo an office hysteroscopy (n = 8). Seventeen women had 26 pregnancies with 19 term deliveries, 1 ectopic pregnancy, 2 abortions, and 4 miscarriages. The clinical courses of the 19 complete gestations were uneventful, but postpartum hemorrhage recurred in 6 women (31.6%) (caused by placenta accreta in 2 women). Fertility and pregnancy outcomes did not differ between women who had undergone embolization versus both embolization and a uterine-sparing surgical procedure.

Recurrence

Placenta accreta recurred in 6 of 21 cases [28.6% (95% CI, 11.3–52.2%)] and was associated with placenta previa in 4 cases. In four of these six cases, the placenta accreta was managed successfully by conservative treatment; in one case it was managed by a cesarean and hysterectomy, and in one case by unsuccessful extirpative treatment followed by a peripartum hysterectomy {Sentilhes, 2010 #482}.

Another series reported recurrence in 27/570 (4.7%, 95% CI 3.0–6.5%) of second and 9/119 (7.6%, 95% CI 2.8–12.3%) of third pregnancies after placenta accreta spectrum in the preceding birth, with an overall recurrence rate of 38/689 (5.5%, 95% CI 3.9–7.5%, compared with the population prevalence of 25.5/10,000 births (95% CI 24.6–26.4) {Baldwin, 2020 #26}.

Summary

PAS rate will continue to escalate in parallel with the ever-increasing rate of uterine procedures. Thereafter, there is more tendency to try conservative surgery than to do hysterectomy. The philosophy behind this is either fertility-preserving or problematic hysterectomy.

So, with passage of time, women healthcare providers encounter more cases who wish either fertility or become pregnant with some possible, although rare, proposed adverse maternal outcomes during pregnancy.

Although the prognosis of subsequent pregnancy after conservative treatment for placenta accreta is found to be mostly fruitful, appropriate preparations should be made to minimize morbidity and mortality resulting from the recurrence of placenta accreta and postpartum hemorrhage. Above all, meticulous counseling of patients of both sides should be done carefully. Pregnancy is possible in most cases of successful conservative management but is associated with an almost 30% risk of PAS disorders in subsequent pregnancies.

References

1. Jauniaux E, et al. FIGO consensus guidelines on placenta accreta spectrum disorders: Epidemiology. Int J Gynaecol Obstet. 2018;140(3):265–73.
2. Irving FC HA. A study of placenta accreta. Surg Gynec Obstet. 1937;64:178–200.
3. Wu S, et al. Abnormal placentation: twenty-year analysis. Am J Obstet Gynecol. 2005;192(5):1458–61.
4. American College of Obstetrics and Gynecology. Obstetric Care Consensus No. 7: Placenta Accreta Spectrum. Obstet Gynecol. 2018;132(6):e259–75.
5. Fox KA, et al. Conservative management of morbidly adherent placenta: expert review. Am J Obstet Gynecol. 2015;213(6):755–60.
6. O'Brien JM, et al. The management of placenta percreta: conservative and operative strategies. Am J Obstet Gynecol. 1996;175(6):1632–8.
7. Muir JC. Conservative treatment of placenta accreta with subsequent normal pregnancy. Am J Obstet Gynecol. 1948;56(4):807.
8. Kabiri D, et al. Outcomes of subsequent pregnancies after conservative treatment for placenta accreta. Int J Gynaecol Obstet. 2014;127(2):206–10.

9. Sentilhes L, et al. Maternal outcome after conservative treatment of placenta accreta. Obstet Gynecol. 2010;115(3):526–34.
10. Clausen C, et al. Management of placenta percreta: a review of published cases. Acta Obstet Gynecol Scand. 2014;93(2):138–43.
11. Jauniaux E, Bhide A. Prenatal ultrasound diagnosis and outcome of placenta previa accreta after cesarean delivery: a systematic review and meta-analysis. Am J Obstet Gynecol. 2017;217(1):27–36.
12. Kutuk MS, et al. Leaving the placenta in situ versus conservative and radical surgery in the treatment of placenta accreta spectrum disorders. Int J Gynaecol Obstet. 2018;140(3):338–44.
13. Palacios-Jaraquemada JM. Diagnosis and management of placenta accreta. Best Pract Res Clin Obstet Gynaecol. 2008;22(6):1133–48.
14. Baldwin HJ, Nippita TA, Torvaldsen S, Ibiebele I, Ford JB, Patterson JA. Outcomes of subsequent births after placenta accreta spectrum. Obstet Gynecol. 2020;136(4):745–55. https://doi.org/10.1097/AOG.0000000000004051. PMID: 32925617.

MIX
Papier aus verantwortungsvollen Quellen
Paper from responsible sources
FSC® C105338

If you have any concerns about our products,
you can contact us on
ProductSafety@springernature.com

In case Publisher is established outside the EU,
the EU authorized representative is:
Springer Nature Customer Service Center GmbH
Europaplatz 3, 69115 Heidelberg, Germany

Printed by Libri Plureos GmbH
in Hamburg, Germany